Use your MIND
To heal your BODY

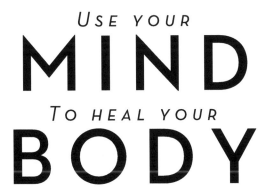

How I used Dr. Sarno's medically proven
treatment plan to eliminate my back pain forever

STEPHEN CONENNA, P.E.

CreateSpace Publishers

Copyright © 2013 by Stephen Conenna.

All rights reserved. No part of this publication may be reproduced, distributed or transmitted in any form or by any means, including photocopying, recording, or other electronic or mechanical methods, without the prior written permission of the publisher, except in the case of brief quotations embodied in critical reviews and certain other noncommercial uses permitted by copyright law. For permission requests, write to the publisher, addressed "Attention: Permissions Coordinator," at the address below.

CreateSpace Publishers
8329 W Sunset Rd Ste 200, Las Vegas, NV 89113-2203

Book Cover by Jesse Alpers
jesse_alpers@me.com

This book is written by a Civil Engineer. The title PE after the author's name stands for Professional Engineer. This book is not written by a physician or health care professional and is not intended as a substitute for medical advice. The reader should consult a physician or health care professional in matters relating to his or her health and particularly with respect to symptoms that may require diagnosis or medical attention.

Publisher's Note: Names, characters, places, and incidents have been changed to protect the privacy of individuals. Any resemblance to actual people, living or dead, or to businesses, companies, events, institutions, or locales is coincidental.

Use Your Mind to Heal Your Body/Stephen Conenna. 1st ed.

Dedicated with deep gratitude to

John E. Sarno, M.D.,
a genius

and

Eric Sherman, Psy.D.,
a gifted psychotherapist.

These men gave me back my life.

All truth passes through three stages.
First, it is ridiculed.
Second, it is violently opposed.
Third, it is accepted as being self-evident.

–Arthur Schopenhauer
German Philosopher
1788-1860

CONTENTS

Acknowledgements

PART I – DISCOVERING MINDBODY MEDICINE

1. Introduction 19
2. What This Book is Not About 23
3. What This Book is About 25
4. How This Book Works – The Power of a Patient's Perspective 33
5. The Beginning of Healing – Discovering What Doesn't Work 37
6. Discovering and Exploring the Inner Terrain 41
7. Unexpected Teachers 51
8. The Aha Moment 59
9. Helping Others Get Better Faster – Creation of the "Alumni Panel" 71

Part II – Applying Mindbody Medicine

10.   Questions and Answers

- Are you saying that this psychosomatic pain is "all in my head" and that I am not really feeling pain? 76
- What was the source of your pain? 76
- How do I know if the source of my pain is psychosomatic or physical? 77
- Have you ever had back pain again or other symptoms, and how do you deal with them? 77
- Did you have to resolve your life circumstances to get rid of the pain? 79
- Did you need to eliminate unconscious repressed emotions to stop the pain? 80
- Do life circumstances still produce rage in you? 81
- Why do I still feel pain if I can, and do, freely express my rage and anger? 82
- I'm doing everything Dr. Sarno says to do, but I still feel pain. What would you do? 84
- What was one of the most challenging aspects of the healing process? 86
- What else can I do to deal with my skepticism? 88

- Dr. Sarno says symptoms are designed to be distractions from unconscious rage. How do you deal with unconscious emotions if they are unconscious? 88

The Nature of the Relationship between Pain and Emotions:
    - I am willing to accept that I have repressed emotions I do not want to feel. Do you mean that the physical pain is a way my body expresses emotional pain? 90
    - Are you saying that I am experiencing symptoms because I may be getting some kind of indirect benefit from having pain? 91
    - What is the relationship between pain and unconscious emotions? 92

- Are you suggesting that I may be inflicting this horrible pain on myself? I am beginning to feel outraged, insulted and offended. I have medical evidence that indicates the source of my pain is physical. 93
- If I accept that the source of my pain is emotional and not physical does that mean that I am defective, or weak in some way? 94
- What is meant by "location substitution" and "symptom imperative"? 96

- What can I do to get better? 98
    - Repudiate the Physical 99
    - Accept the Psychological 99
    - The Daily Reminders 100
    - The Daily Study Program 101
    - The Treasure Map Process 103

- Are you implying that all back surgery is unnecessary? 114

- Almost every book I've read on the subject of back pain has back exercises. Do they help? 115

- I have been working with a psychotherapist for many years. Why do I still have pain? 116

- In addition to Dr. Sarno's work, does peer-reviewed medical literature exist regarding the psychosomatic treatment of pain? 116

- Why has psychosomatic diagnosis and treatment not received more attention and recognition from mainstream medicine? 118

Part III – Your Role

11. Ending Pain Forever 123

Recommended References 130
Recent Research in the Field of Mindbody Medicine 133
Thank You Dr. Sarno Project 141
Endnotes 145

ACKNOWLEDGEMENTS

A miracle is never lost. It may touch many people you have not even met, and produce undreamed of changes in situations of which you are not even aware.

—A Course In Miracles

Dr. Sarno and Eric—you have made your life's work be about others. Those who you have touched have touched others, and so on, and the world is a healthier, happier place thanks to you.

Dad, Mom, San, Bet and Jen—through you and your families I know love and I know joy.

My Landmark family—you never stopped seeing the possibility of this book making the difference it is intended to make in the world. You are inspiration itself.

Thank you Ruth Antrich—you not only provided professional and impeccable proofreading skills, you lent powerful encouragement through the final stages of birthing this book. Jennifer Hamady, Alex Forbes and Beth Warren—I so appreciate the valuable time to carefully read every word of the manuscript and golden feedback you provided. Brian Cousin—thank you for being the best friend anyone could ask for.

Jeffrey Mironov, my brother—you demonstrate, "*When I forget who I am, I serve you; when I remember who I am, I am you.*"¹ I am forever grateful.

As all who contributed know, the purpose of this book is to end chronic pain. To the extent we accomplish this, know that we did so together.

Based on my experience of many years in dealing with back pain what Mr. Conenna has written about this disorder is very much in tune with my concepts of cause and treatment.

I recommend this highly.

—JOHN E. SARNO, M.D.
September 28, 2012

PART I

DISCOVERING MINDBODY MEDICINE

ONE

INTRODUCTION

I am in the prime of my life. Having graduated from Columbia University's School of Engineering and Applied Science, I am now the owner and operator of an engineering and construction firm, working shoulder to shoulder with laborers, jack-hammering concrete. Suddenly I hear a pop in my lower back. A jolt of pain races from my lower back down my left leg into the second to last toe of my foot, leaving a trail of burning pain. Every step I take on my left leg is torturous. Months and years pass as I tolerate agonizing pain day and night, wondering if I will ever live normally again.

After two years of countless, ineffective visits to medical doctors and alternative practitioners, I discovered and was treated by Dr. John E. Sarno, a professor of rehabilitation medicine and attending physician at the Rusk Institute for Rehabilitation at New York University Medical Center in New York City. I have now been

INTRODUCTION

pain-free for over ten years. Deeply indebted for the life-altering impact Dr. Sarno had on me, I am committed to using my experiences and what I learned to help other people who are suffering from similar maladies.

Dr. Sarno, in his *New York Times* best selling book, *Healing Back Pain* asserts that for years, millions of Americans have been misdiagnosed as having pain with a physical basis, when in fact they are suffering from psychosomatic (synonymous with mindbody) disorders. This ongoing misdiagnosis has led to the epidemic spread of chronic pain syndromes, perpetuating needless suffering, and rendered our health care system in a state of crisis. Recent medical research is now beginning to substantiate this. I believe it is a duty and privilege for patients such as myself, who have gotten better by applying mindbody medical principles, to make their healing experiences known to fellow sufferers, the medical community and society at large so as to reverse this alarming and devastating trend.

While Dr. Sarno has written extensively about the principles and practice of psychosomatic medicine from a *clinician's point of view*, the purpose of this book is to complement his work with a *patient's perspective* about what it takes to deal with and recover from psychosomatic illness. This is not meant to be a substitute for Dr. Sarno's groundbreaking efforts, rather, a unique and vital supplement that only a patient who has recovered from a psychosomatic disorder can provide.

This book may also serve as a stand-alone primer to mindbody medicine. As you begin to understand the relationship between real physical pain and emotions, you will get to the root cause of your pain condition and eliminate it forever.

> "Information is the penicillin that cures this disorder."[2]
> —Dr. Sarno

You will find important information here, essential insights and a clear look into the distinct type of thinking required on the part of a patient to overcome mindbody ailments so that you can successfully eliminate your pain in the least amount of time possible.

If a critical mass of people, together with the support of modern physicians, begins to heal themselves of these heinous maladies through the power and efficacy of mindbody medicine, we can stop the spread of pain epidemics, restore integrity to our health care system and put an end to the needless suffering of millions.

TWO

WHAT THIS BOOK IS NOT ABOUT

This book is *not* about:

- Alternative Medicine
- Back Exercises
- Biofeedback
- Body Work
- Breathing Techniques
- Chiropractic
- Diet, Nutrition or Supplements
- Energy Work
- Hands-on Healing
- Hypnosis
- Injections
- Magnet Therapy
- Massage
- Mental Imagery

WHAT THIS BOOK IS NOT ABOUT

- New Age Medicine
- Physical Therapy
- Positive Thinking
- Prescription Medication or Over-the-Counter Drugs
- Relaxation
- Spine Strengthening
- Stress Management
- Stress Reduction
- Stretching
- Surgery
- Visualization
- Yoga

This book is not an attack, incrimination or an attempt to disprove or discredit any of these modalities or techniques. People have gotten relief using many of these methods. This book is simply not about any of them.

This book is a unique, groundbreaking and comprehensive approach to diagnosing and treating chronic pain. By uncovering the *root cause* of many physical pain conditions, that is, the primary role that emotions play in causing illness, theses symptoms can be eliminated once and for all—without drugs, surgery or physical therapy.

THREE

WHAT THIS BOOK IS ABOUT

*There are a thousand hacking at the branches...
to one who is striking at the root.*

— HENRY DAVID THOREAU
Walden

This book is about psychosomatic medicine.

The Merriam-Webster dictionary defines "psychosomatic" as "bodily symptoms caused by mental or emotional factors." Therefore:

> Psychosomatic Medicine is the treatment of real, physical, bodily symptoms by psychological means.

Unfortunately, in common everyday usage, the term, "psychosomatic" mistakenly implies "imaginary" or "all in the head." This is a medically incorrect use of the

WHAT THIS BOOK IS ABOUT

word. This book discusses the treatment of real, genuine, pain *whose source is psychological.*

The book is about treating real pain based on the innovative medical methodology pioneered by Dr. John E. Sarno, a Professor of Clinical Rehabilitation Medicine at the NYU School of Medicine and an attending physician at the Rusk Institute of Rehabilitation Medicine/NYU Medical Center for nearly fifty years from 1965 to 2012. Beginning in 1982 with the publication of *"Mind Over Back Pain,"*[3] the first of several books authored on the subject, Dr. Sarno developed the diagnosis and treatment of TMS (Tension Myoneural Syndrome.) According to Dr. Sarno, **TMS "is a benign (though painful) physiologic aberration of soft tissue (not the spine), and is caused by an emotional process."**[4] That is, TMS is a harmless, though painful, condition that causes real pain in the back, legs, shoulders, neck, and other areas of the body. "In this condition, the brain orders a reduction of blood flow to a specific part of the body, resulting in mild oxygen deprivation, which causes pain and other symptoms, depending on what tissues have been oxygen deprived."[5] **Therefore, since the root cause of the pain is emotional, it can and must be treated psychologically.**

Based on thousands of case histories, Dr. Sarno concluded that, "The pain, stiffness, burning pressure, numbness, tingling and weakness were caused by mild oxygen deprivation in the muscles, nerves or tendons involved in each case. In itself this was harmless.

> "Although it could produce more severe pain than anything else I knew of in clinical medicine, you would not be left with residual damage when your symptoms disappeared."[6]
> —Dr. Sarno

Dr. Sarno's discovery was and, unfortunately, remains a radical departure from the traditional, conventional treatment of back pain and other equivalent pain disorders. The most distinguishing feature of this new diagnosis is that it works. Consistent, numerically impressive therapeutic success is more than a reasonable test of validity and proof of the accuracy of this diagnosis. In more than 40 years of Dr. Sarno's clinical practice, over 10,000 patients, most of whom have been rendered pain-free and fully physically active, have recovered simply by learning about the psychology, physiology and treatment of mindbody syndromes.[7]

While many people, including myself, consider Dr. Sarno to be a medical genius, in a sense, he is simply a doctor who had the courage to tell the truth. For nine years, early on in his practice as a family physician, he

WHAT THIS BOOK IS ABOUT

made conventional diagnoses such as back sprain, muscle pull, weak muscles, various spinal disorders, narrowed disk spaces, or sciatica. He prescribed bed rest, muscle relaxants, analgesics (pain killers), physical therapy, ultrasound, ice packs, deep heat, massage, and steroid injections. He trained people about how to bend and lift properly. "The results of such treatment were poor and unpredictable; my practice was frustrating and unfulfilling. Failure was inevitable because I didn't know what I was dealing with."[8]

Then, in a flash of inspiration, Dr. Sarno noticed a remarkable trend among his patients: almost all of them had a history of one or more psychosomatic manifestations in the course of their lives—it dawned on him that their very physical complaints could also be psychosomatic.[9] When Dr. Sarno started treating his patients using the principles and practice of psychosomatic medicine, the results were "almost immediate."[10] Dr. Sarno explains that this mindbody methodology continues be effective to this day, over 40 years later, because he has uncovered the real source of much chronic pain.

Dr. Sarno's breakthrough was *not* simply a "new approach" to the treatment of back pain. That is, it was not a new way to treat the "physical causes" of back pain. This was a "new *diagnosis*." Dr. Sarno recounts, "I told my patients there was nothing wrong with their backs. I explained that they had a harmless condition that must be treated through the mind, not the body. Awareness, insight, knowledge and information were the magic medicines that would cure this disorder—and nothing else could do it."[11]

> *"I don't treat pain! That would be symptomatic treatment and it's poor medicine. I treat the disorder that is the root cause of the pain."*[12]
> —Dr. Sarno

Inside this book you will gain awareness, insight and information from the perspective of a patient who has successfully gone from having incapacitating pain to being pain free. You will learn what the process was like for me and how to overcome your own doubts, skepticism, fears, and insecurities so as to deal powerfully with the inevitable ups and downs of recovery. I will describe in plain language what I learned about *why* a part of the mind feels the need to cause such debilitating pain. Armed with a clear understanding of the relationship between your emotions and your pain, you will be able to eliminate your pain for good.

A few words about terminology. In line with Dr. Sarno, throughout the book I use the words *psychosomatic* and *mindbody* interchangeably.[13] TMS (Ten-

WHAT THIS BOOK IS ABOUT

sion Mysositis Syndrome) is also used as a shortcut for psychosomatic pain. Psychophysiologic disorder is another term for real pain that is psychologically induced that is being used by current researchers. Finally, Dr. Sarno joins the words *mind* and *body* in honor of the clear connection between emotions and the body[14] and I have followed suit.

In summarizing what this book is about, it is essential to understand that numerous widespread physical disorders, some having reached epidemic levels, serve the same purpose as back pain. That is, "they are designed to be distractions from unconscious rage."[15] Therefore, they can and should be dealt with in the same way as back pain: psychologically.

Below is a partial list of other psychosomatic disorders that are commonly attributed to structural abnormalities or other physical phenomena.[16] Please brace yourself as you may be shocked and angered by what you read. Keep in mind that if the true cause of these devastating disorders were known by mainstream medicine, they would not have reached their current catastrophic levels.

EQUIVALENTS

- Acne, hives
- Allergies

- Asthma
- Carpal tunnel syndrome
- Dizziness
- Eczema
- Esophagospasm
- Fibromyalgia
- Gastroesophageal reflux
- Hay fever
- Hiatus hernia
- Irritable Bowel Syndrome
- Knee Tendonitis
- Migraine headache
- Most cases of prostatitus and sexual dysfunction
- OCD (obsessive-compulsive disorder)
- Peptic ulcer
- Pre-ulcer states
- Prostatitis
- Psoriasis
- Shoulder Tendonitis
- Spastic colon
- Tennis Elbow
- Tension headache
- Tinnitus (ringing in the ears)
- Vertigo

The same methodology I used to treat my back pain applies perfectly to any of these maladies. Since these

WHAT THIS BOOK IS ABOUT

ailments serve the same purpose as most chronic back, neck and leg pain, that is, to distract attention from unconscious emotions, they are frequently referred to as "equivalents." Of course, with any of these disorders it is important to consult your regular physician and rule out any serious disease.

FOUR

HOW THIS BOOK WORKS – THE POWER OF A PATIENT'S PERSPECTIVE

*You cannot teach a man anything;
you can only help him find it within himself.*

— GALILEO GALILEI
Italian Astronomer and Physicist
(1564-1642)

After a brief chronology of when my pain started and what I did to get better, the heart of this book follows in a "Question and Answer" format.

While medical evaluation and treatment is indispensable to someone in pain, a successful patient's perspective is an invaluable and often overlooked treatment asset. This is particularly the case when dealing with psychosomatic disorders because in mindbody treatment a great deal of responsibility is placed on the patient.

HOW THIS BOOK WORKS

Traditional (non-psychosomatic) treatment commonly involves a doctor giving injections, performing surgery, or prescribing pharmaceuticals—all reducing a patient's active role. In the case of psychosomatic medical treatment, doctors can only lead the way to recovery. It is up to the patient to follow. As we have said, when psychosomatic illness is the diagnosis, information is the prescription. A patient must then actively take the information presented and incorporate it into his or her life. This type of treatment is not only "more knowledge;" the patient must learn to *think differently* and *apply* that knowledge.

Two particular types of different thinking will be required of you. First, you must learn to *think psychologically, not physically*. Second, you must learn to think about your *unconscious emotions*. Of course, this begs the question, how can I think about unconscious emotions if they are unconscious?

The "Question and Answer" format that follows is designed to assist the reader in both of these respects. You will go inside the mind of a patient as he learns to think differently. Observing how someone else discovers, confronts and deals with uncomfortable emotions provides a safe and effective model for a person to learn *how* to think differently for oneself.

Seeing hidden emotions in someone else can be a valuable gateway into seeing one's own hidden emotions. You may recognize thoughts, feelings and experiences in your own psychology that were once hidden from your view. You may not have been aware of these emotions because—as you will see with ever-increasing clarity—a part of your mind works to distract your attention from these painful emotions.

Dr. Sarno's research indicates that psychosomatic pain "is created in order to distract the attention of the sufferer from what is going on in the emotional sphere. It is intended to focus one's attention on the body *instead* of the mind. It is a response to the need to keep those terrible, antisocial, unkind, childish, angry, selfish feelings...from becoming conscious."[17] Having identified the source of the pain, treatment becomes clear:

> *Since the purpose of psychosomatic pain is to distract you from what your mind fears are unbearable emotions, when you confront and accept these emotions, the pain no longer serves a purpose and disappears.*

FIVE

THE BEGINNING OF HEALING – DISCOVERING WHAT DOESN'T WORK

For two years following my construction incident, I became consumed with finding a cure for my back pain. I hobbled in agony from one medical appointment to another. If you lifted up my shirt and looked at my spinal column, instead of an up and down line you would see that severe muscle spasms were pulling my lower spine diagonally to the left. Physical therapists recommended physical therapy, chiropractors recommended chiropractics, and back surgeons recommended back surgery.

Prior to the construction incident, I had a 15-year history of intermittent back pain that began as an undergraduate student in engineering school. Sometimes my back would simply hurt for a few days or weeks. Other times, I would be bedridden. When I was bedridden, it wasn't that I didn't *want* to get out of bed; I physically

THE BEGINNING OF HEALING

could not get out of bed. Interestingly, as debilitating as the pain was, it would eventually disappear as if I never had it. This time, however, the pain would not go away. An MRI identified disk herniations at the L4-L5 and L5-S1 inter-vertebral locations of my lumbar spine. When I heard the results of the MRI, I became frightened that something had been irreparably damaged. I feared that I was going to be in pain for the rest of my life, and people in my life were deeply concerned.

As I mentioned, I'm a Columbia University graduate and a civil engineer, so I've learned to rely on my intellect and I tried to figure my way out of this painful situation. I tried everything. Orthopedic doctors diagnosed me with sciatica and prescribed painkillers and physical therapy. Physical therapy was like going to a torture chamber. I was literally put on a rack, with my upper-body strapped to one end of a machine, my feet to another, and pulled apart! I had traditional acupuncture and I also had the type of acupuncture in which they electrify the needles. I visited numerous chiropractors who provided temporary relief, but they were all ineffective over time. A shiatsu masseuse once left me black and blue after a deep tissue treatment, stuck a leaf on my back and asked me to come back in two weeks! I even purchased an inversion machine where I hung upside down for hours! That actually provided temporary relief because, to my engineering mind, this would reverse the compressive forces on the vertebrae that were causing my disks to bulge and impinge on my sciatic nerve. Since it made sense on paper, I actually felt better—while hanging upside down. Of course, once I got back on my feet, the pain returned. It's easy to make light of all of this now, but I remember how desperate I was to find a cure and how terrified I was that nothing would work.

I went to a major medical school library and intensely researched chronic back pain, herniated disks, and sciatica. I read physiology books, journals, and research papers. I studied charts, data, and case study MRIs, some of which looked frighteningly like my own MRI. Being an engineer, I was able to read my MRI, given its similarity to a blueprint. The disk bulge was undeniable. I could identify the extrusion and even the point where it impinged on my sciatic nerve. The more I learned about back pain mechanics, the more I bought into the structural diagnosis. I was becoming hopeless and feeling more pain.

My research included bookstores. I read just about every back pain book on the shelves. They all echoed the same theme I found in medical texts: "a structural anatomic defect is causing the pain." I found a singular and notable exception to this diagnosis in one thin, little book, which I had discovered early on in my research. When I picked up this book, strangely titled, "Mind Over

THE BEGINNING OF HEALING

Back Pain," by Dr. John Sarno I thought to myself, "How unusual! What connection can there possibly be between my mind and a structural condition?" I skimmed through it in the bookstore, and I said to myself, "Oh my God! Who is this misguided doctor who seems to be saying that the pain is all in my head? My pain is real! I can barely walk. I can't do the things that I want to do. Look at the nonsense that people are buying these days!" Angrily, I threw the book down and continued on with my search for a cure.

SIX

DISCOVERING AND EXPLORING THE INNER TERRAIN

> *Direct your eye right inward, and you'll find a thousand regions in your mind yet undiscovered. Travel them, and be expert in home-cosmography.*
>
> — Henry David Thoreau
> Walden

Two years later, I had exhausted every non-invasive treatment option I knew of and was headed towards surgery. As a last resort, I tried epidural steroid injections. I was wheeled into an operating room and doctors injected cortisone into my spine. After the first injection, the pain went away and I was so elated that I literally ran around my block thinking, "I'm free! I'm free!" Two weeks later, I was back to the same level of pain as before the shot. I underwent five more injections. With each epidural, the relief period dimin-

DISCOVERING AND EXPLORING THE INNER TERRAIN

ished, and eventually they made no difference at all. Oral steroids did not work either.

Desperate, I went to see a back surgeon who recommended surgery. At the bottom of his report it said, *literally in fine print*, that there is no guarantee that the surgery will relieve the pain, that I may need future surgery and possibly bone grafts, and that the procedure might result in death! This, together with reading that permanent nerve damage may result if I refused surgery, threw me into an absolute panic. While surgery seemed to be my only remaining option, my research on back surgery was filled with contradictions and inconsistencies. I met people in physical therapy who were recovering *from surgery*—months after the surgery! Surgeons told them that, while the disk problem was "cured," scar tissue resulting from the surgical procedure was now causing the pain. I met *some* people who got better from surgery, but not everyone. Some people were worse off.

I began to become skeptical about the structural diagnosis. I read about cases where a disk herniation was on one side of the spine and the pain radiated down the *other* leg. That didn't make any sense at all. In my own life, when I tried yoga to relieve the pain, I couldn't understand why I was able to do certain strenuous postures and movements *in class* without pain, but would then have pain *after class*. Also, when the pain first began, it hurt when I *lay* down, and I would get relief when I *sat* down. Then, after reading a report that showed that inter-vertebral stress increases when one sits, *the pain shifted* and it began to hurt when I *sat* down, and I would get relief when I *lay* down. I asked myself, "If the herniation is consistent, why is the pain pattern inconsistent? Why does it come and go? Why does it hurt when I do certain things and not others? If the cause is simply structural, why are there so many people who don't get better after back surgery?"

The other part of the structural diagnosis story that didn't add up was that four years *prior* to my construction incident, I had another extended attack of back pain that began while on vacation shortly after ending a six-year romantic relationship. Although the pain went away after a few months, during treatment I had an MRI which indicated disk herniations at L4-L5, L5-S1. The problem was that the doctor who examined my *current* MRIs, after *four years* of being pain free, observed that the herniations had not changed at all! The technical term for this is "no interval change" which was written in the findings of the new MRI report. I thought to myself, "How could I have been pain free during those four years even though the disk herniations were there the whole time? I also thought, "If I got better without surgery then, why should I need surgery now?"

Desperate to make sure I exhausted every possible treatment option, I remembered that thin, little book I *skimmed* years ago having something to do with mind and back pain. I rushed to a bookstore hoping I could find it since I did not remember the title or author. Fortunately, I found a newer edition of the book, *Healing Back Pain: The Mindbody Connection,*" by Dr. John Sarno—and this time I *read* it. What I read startled me. The author *never* said that the pain is all in my mind or imaginary. He said that the pain is real and, in fact, one of the most painful symptoms in medicine. The *source* of the pain is one's mind. The pain is *not* due to a disk abnormality, even though one may be present. His book referenced a 1994 study in the *New England Journal of Medicine*:

> *A 1994 scientific research study showed that over two thirds of people <u>without</u> pain had disk abnormalities.*[18]
> —New England Journal of Medicine

Since the importance of this finding must not be missed, I will repeat it: *over two thirds* of people <u>without</u> pain had disk abnormalities. At first, I was shocked that none of the medical literature I researched referenced this article. Upon closer reflection, it stands to reason that anyone focusing on disk abnormalities a principle source of pain would need to overlook this study. I began to understand why there were so many inconsistencies with the structural diagnosis.

> *Disk abnormalities, like other structural abnormalities found on X-rays, CT scans or MRIs are normal changes associated with activity and aging. They do not lead to pain.* [19]
> —Dr. Sarno

As I read Dr. Sarno's description of his typical patients (see below), my personal traits leapt off the pages. The typical personality characteristics of mindbody patients are listed below. See if your personality type makes you a candidate for psychosomatic pain.

PERSONALITY TRAITS ASSESSMENT

There are 3 main factors that create the environment for mindbody pain to arise: your childhood, your present circumstances and your personality. The questions below may be used to asses your if your personality has

DISCOVERING AND EXPLORING THE INNER TERRAIN

a tendency to accumulate *internal* stress and therefore manifest psychosomatic pain.

For each of the personality traits below rate yourself from 1 being "I disagree" to 5 being "I agree."

1. I have a great sense of responsibility
   disagree 1 2 3 4 5 *agree*

2. I am hard-working
   disagree 1 2 3 4 5 *agree*

3. I am a perfectionist—I try to do the right thing all the time
   disagree 1 2 3 4 5 *agree*

4. I am a "good-ist"—I'm driven to be good all the time
   disagree 1 2 3 4 5 *agree*

5. I put more pressure on yourself than anyone else
   disagree 1 2 3 4 5 *agree*

6. I am self-motivated
   disagree 1 2 3 4 5 *agree*

7. I am self-disciplined
   disagree 1 2 3 4 5 *agree*

8. I am my own worst critic
   disagree 1 2 3 4 5 *agree*

9. There's nothing I can't handle
   disagree 1 2 3 4 5 *agree*

10. I have a strong inner drive to succeed in both business and family matters
    disagree 1 2 3 4 5 agree

11. I need to be loved, admired, respected
    disagree 1 2 3 4 5 agree

12. I have a tendency towards guilt
    disagree 1 2 3 4 5 agree

13. I am a worrier
    disagree 1 2 3 4 5 agree

Total Score: _____

Results

26-38: *Moderate likelihood for psychosomatic pain*
39-52: *Strong likelihood for psychosomatic pain*
53-65: *Very Strong likelihood for psychosomatic pain*

....

I was startled. I said, "That's me!" This is when the penny dropped. Instantly I saw how I, or anyone with these traits, would accumulate enormous volumes of internal stress and how it could grow exponentially. For example, by always being good, at some level I expect people to always be good in return. When inevitably they are not, I become outraged. Now, here is where the

DISCOVERING AND EXPLORING THE INNER TERRAIN

rage (and corresponding pain) increases exponentially: I cannot express, or even acknowledge this internal state to myself, because—*that wouldn't be good!* Even though I would subsequently go through a year of psychotherapy, as well as dozens of small group sessions with Dr. Sarno, before I became completely pain-free, I knew at that moment that I had found my answer.

I made an appointment with Dr. Sarno, which accomplished two critical steps. First, he confirmed that there was nothing physically wrong with my back by ruling out fractures, infections, tumors, cancer, bone disease, and other serious disorders. Second, he diagnosed me with a psychosomatic disorder known as Tension Myositis Syndrome (TMS).

> *"Tension Myositis Syndrome (TMS) is a painful condition in which the brain orders a reduction of blood flow to a specific part of the body, resulting in mild oxygen deprivation, which causes pain and other symptoms."*[20]
> —Dr. Sarno

Committed to eliminating the pain as soon as possible, I began to see a psychotherapist recommended by

Dr. Sarno. I had the great fortune to work with Dr. Eric Sherman, a gifted psychotherapist who, I can honestly say, saved my life. Over the course of my year-long treatment, I had moments when I was completely pain free, and also had moments when I would regress to being in as much pain as when I started.

What happened next was completely unanticipated. I was ushered into a world that I thought I knew, but was, in fact, foreign to me: the world of feelings and emotions, or the *inner terrain*. In this new world new laws applied, many of which ran counter to my familiar laws of logic and physics. In this realm, loving and hating the same person at the same time easily coexists; you can have murderous thoughts and maintain innocence. I entered into a period where I experienced tremendous emotional relief. As I began to understand myself, the burden of shameful, disowned baggage swept under the rug of consciousness lightened. I was becoming fully expressive and I felt lighter and happier.

SEVEN

UNEXPECTED TEACHERS

I was determined to get maximum value from psychotherapy (especially since it was a significant out-of-pocket expense) so, after each session I would go to a nearby coffee shop and write notes about what my therapist and I discussed. Inevitably, this would spark a chain of thoughts regarding different areas of my life and I would think and write about those areas in ways I had never done before.

In addition to therapy, I was regularly attending Dr. Sarno's weekly Group Sessions for three or four months. The Group Sessions were a vital part of our treatment program. Gathered in a circle in one of the medical classrooms at the NYU Medical Center on the East Side of Manhattan, Dr. Sarno would lead twenty to thirty active patients, in a revelatory conversation. Patients were mostly middle- to upper-class, articulate, educated New Yorkers who, on the surface, appeared to have it all together. There was a tanned business man in a sharp pin-striped suit, a housewife with manicured nails and perfect blonde highlights, a stately Hassid in traditional attire, a grandfatherly-like gentleman with a gold-tipped walking stick, and a young, new mother of twins, to describe a few.

With little regard to his obvious back pain, Dr. Sarno engaged Walter, the elegant grandfather. We learned that he was mourning the loss of his wife of fifty years, Martha. Intelligent and sensitive, the elderly gentleman could not understand why he was in pain since he was clearly in touch with his feelings of grief and sadness.

Dr. Sarno asked, "Walter, who are you angry at?"

A bit taken aback, Walter answered, "Life—it's not fair that good people die. He thought a bit more, "I wish Martha was with me now."

The old man was nearly un-confrontable. That is, one would have to be heartless to challenge Walter's reasons for emotional pain and suffering. That's when Dr. Sarno dropped a bomb which resulted in a deafening silence across what seemed to be the entire East Side: "Walter, I want you to consider, that you are angry with Martha—for leaving you."

The elegant blonde removed her silk scarf and Walter wept.

With divine-like compassion, Dr. Sarno turned to us and explained that these are the emotions of which psychosomatic disorders are made. Clearly, it would be utterly selfish, heartless and even cruel for Walter to feel anger toward his deceased wife. The pain that had been distracting Walter day and night, served masterfully, albeit duplicitously, to keep these impermissible feelings hidden. Of course, feeling resentful towards people who leave us is also human and inescapable.

Walter composed himself. "Yes. I can see that I've been angry at Martha. And I can see that this doesn't mean that I love her any less."

Walter walked out of that session upright, brandishing his walking stick which was now more of an accessory than a cane. He seemed approachable and any airs of social privilege had vanished. No longer needing to act dignified to cover self-loathing, Walter had reclaimed his self worth and personal dignity.

We all walked out a bit more upright that evening.

We learned that Cindy, the blonde housewife, was experiencing excruciating neck pain. We were simultaneously envious and disgusted by her "problem" of having to deal with several hundred-thousand dollar home renovations and unreliable contractors. In a short time, we learn that Cindy married into money. With her mother and sisters still struggling to make ends meet, she discovers that she feels that she does not have the right to feel angry and frustrated over what should be petty and frivolous issues. Cindy breathes a sigh of re-

UNEXPECTED TEACHERS

lief, "My issues are my issues and they don't make me a stuck-up snob." We all laugh together—mostly at the comedic tragedy of our own self-assessments.

Yacov, the Hassid, has been dealing with painful abdominal cramps and diarrhea that has been diagnosed as Irritable Bowl Syndrome. His symptoms began nearly two years ago, one month after the tragic stillborn death of his daughter. He shares with us that he is ashamed of wishing that she had never been conceived and acknowledges that, even though he can't feel the rage, he must be mad at God. As Yacov embraces all of his emotions, a deep sense of compassion for our humanity comes over all of us.

To this day I remain humbled, and profoundly inspired by the generosity these unexpected teachers who bared their fears, pain and insecurities. I was moved by every patient's courage to pursue this treatment in the face of little evidence of its efficacy. Perhaps it was courage, or maybe it was that everything else had failed. Many patients had failed surgery, some multiple surgeries. Listening to Dr. Sarno speak and interact with us was like being with a wise man. He stood there, stoic, in a crisp staff-length white coat, commanding, authoritative, penetrative and insightful, yet completely compassionate and always the consummate medical professional.

> "There nothing wrong with your back!"
>
> "Don't think structurally, think emotionally!"
>
> "Get mad at your brain, give it hell!"
>
> "Your symptoms are a trick your mind is playing on you—don't fall for it!"
>
> —DR. SARNO

Yet, even though every aspect of the treatment program was making intellectual sense to me and I was feeling better emotionally – which is to say that I was feeling lighter, less stressed, feeling better about my life and what was possible – I was still in pain. Something was missing.

I wanted to meet someone who had been through Dr. Sarno's program and became pain-free. I wanted to *see* that it was possible to get better and what life looked like after treatment.

One day, after a session, while sitting in the coffee shop with my well-worn, dog-eared, highlighted copy of Dr. Sarno's book, a woman approached me and said, "I noticed your book—are you a patient of Dr. Sarno?" I didn't know it at the time, but that chance encounter would be a pivotal moment in my treatment and would affect hundreds of other people as well.

The woman introduced herself as Sue, and went on to share her story with me. "I was a patient of Dr. Sarno. I was bedridden for four months. I thought my life was ruined." She shared that over the course of her 20-year marriage to Scott, he matured from a verbally hostile, short tempered, difficult spouse into the loving, affectionate husband Sue always envisioned. When Scott lost his well-paying job and chose to take a weekend position in order to pursue his art work and be able to drive the kids to and from school, Sue's dreams of getting out of debt and buying a home seemed to be dashed. It seemed to her that Scott was being lazy and selfish. That's when she developed severely incapacitating leg pain. What emerged in her work with Dr. Sarno was that the source of her pain was a profound sense of guilt for being angry at Scott who is now loving and kind towards her and the kids. She accepted these emotions as part of being human and became pain-free within weeks. Seven years later, Sue remains free of pain.

I thank her for her openness and then I shared my story. She encouraged me to keep doing what I was doing and assured me that I would soon be well.

> It occurred to me that patients who had been through treatment and are now pain-free could expedite the healing process for other patients.

I was profoundly moved and inspired by Sue's story. All the sharing from the Group Sessions came together. I saw the future and in that future I was pain-free. In that moment, I decided that when I got better, I would find a way to provide that same living possibility and inspiration for other people.

EIGHT

THE AHA MOMENT

Meeting Sue and participating in the Group Sessions were beginning to affect me. I was undergoing a shift that went beyond intellectual or conceptual understanding. The possibility that I was *not* permanently damaged, that there was *not* something physically wrong with me, and that I *could* be pain-free for the rest of my life was beginning to take root. This understanding was becoming a "knowing" rather than merely an idea that made sense.

At this time, I had a great realization. I became aware that there are *two distinct steps* to the process of looking at one's emotions and healing psychosomatic pain. In other words, my *Aha Moment* was realizing that there are <u>two stages</u> to the *Aha Moment*. First, there's the "Ah" when you have an insight, or think something that you had not previously considered. Then, there's the "Ha," where you deepen that insight and the healing happens. I will

THE AHA MOMENT

clarify this below, using my life, circumstances and personal history as an example.

Before I share my own experiences, I want to emphasize that there may not have been major traumatic events in our younger years for us to accumulate a significant amount of disowned feelings. Even though subtle and usually unintended, childhood incidents can be impactful and enduring, with significant psychological fallout relegated to the unconscious. The acknowledgment, validation and legitimization of *whatever* feelings we experience, especially during childhood, is the key to overcoming psychosomatic pain.

For me, the first stage, or "Ah," begins in Buenos Aires, Argentina where I was born to loving parents of Italian descent. My father is a silver-haired man with an Italian accent. He's charming, funny, gracious, and if you met him, you would *love* him. The problem was that a part of me *hated* him—and prior to therapy I could *never* have said that to anybody, *including myself.*

When we immigrated from to New York City, Dad worked two jobs while mom stayed at home with my three sisters and me. Dad mostly played the role of provider and disciplinarian, while mom took care of us kids. Dad's main priority was our family's safety and wellbeing. He worked hard so that we could eventually move out of our small apartment and into our own home. I had a classic Italian upbringing and our family's closeness was often envied by my friends. We never lacked for any basic necessities and I knew I was loved and cared for. Nevertheless, this upbringing was, for me, an emotional double-edged sword.

For example, in our home, dinner was sacred and missing it was not an option. While it was clearly a rich opportunity to share our lives with each other, laugh and grow up together—as a child, it often occurred to me as a burden or obligation. After all, my friends were allowed to miss dinner and play or watch TV. But, if I so much as arrived late, reprimand was delivered surely and swiftly.

Dad never missed a day of work and kept long work hours, accepting every overtime opportunity he was offered—even if it meant working long past midnight. While I missed his companionship and at one level resented that he was not available much to play and spend time together, I was at the same time glad not to encounter the disciplinarian.

Dad's basic philosophy was old-school and conservative: "best not to take any unnecessary risks." Dad insisted on keeping us kids close to home; I was not allowed to participate in organized sports or attend a specialized out-of-area high school like I wanted. Also, my ambitious projects (such as starting a business or moving away from home) were met with opposition and apparent hostility. When he would say that he was doing this because "he loved me" it only added to my confusion and inner-conflict.

Loud arguments between dad and mom or between dad and my younger sisters would erupt without warning. I became their advocate, a skilled mediator and diplomat. In this capacity, I learned that my emotions, particularly anger and resentment, were a liability, so repressing them became an effective, and eventually automatic defense mechanism. Being a good boy, agreeable and well behaved also worked well to keep me out of trouble with dad.

Of course, prior to therapy, I couldn't articulate any of this. I couldn't allow myself to have any of those feelings because, as a good Italian boy, you *gotta love your dad!* I couldn't understand why, whenever I was in the same room as him, I was uneasy, annoyed and edgy. In therapy—and this is the "Ah"—I discovered an entire reservoir of anger and rage towards my father that I had not been aware of or "owned." In therapy I saw, felt and understood my rage. I realized, "Wow, I am *really* furious. I'm actually enraged." I didn't know it was there before, and now I see that it's there. It's there because this thing happened in my childhood, and that thing happened when I went to college, and another thing happened when I moved out of my parents' home, and so on." I could now see the rage, explain the rage, and even feel the rage. I validated and legitimized the rage. As a result,

I felt better emotionally—I had a sense of freedom—but I still had pain. So, the "Ah" insight is a great start, but alone it's <u>not</u> going to get you better.

Since simply understanding or even feeling my rage didn't resolve the pain, I thought, "I am going to express this rage to my father and get rid of it." I told my therapist what I planned to do and he said, "Wait a minute." Then, he made one of those statements that you hear and never forget for the rest of your life: "Steve, this work is an *inside job*." The earth seemed to have stood still. At that moment, I knew viscerally that the work of my healing was internal—between me and me—and had *nothing* to do with my father.

I learned that what was causing my pain had to do with how I felt *about myself* for having those feelings about my own father. I saw what I was thinking: "What kind of miserable, thankless, ungrateful, traitorous, betraying son has these kinds of feelings towards his *own father*? My father loves me; he would do *anything* for me. He would die for me." In therapy, I discovered that it is OK, and in fact human, to have rage and resentment towards people I love—*completely human!* All my life I suppressed those feelings. It was intolerable for me to have those feelings. It was unbearable and impermissible for me to have those feelings. Pain distracted me from those feelings. Pain protected me from this unbearable distress. To a part of my mind, it was preferable to spend twenty-four hours a day, seven days a week, month after month, year after year, painfully limping from one physical therapist to a chiropractor to another guy sticking needles in me, than to feel the self-loathing of a man who hates his father *and shouldn't.*

When I learned that it's all right, and in fact *normal*, to have bad[1] feelings, I no longer needed to use pain to distract or protect myself from these emotions. *That* was the "Ha." My therapist said, "You know Steve, I'd be concerned for you if you *didn't* have those feelings." What a load off my back! As it became OK for me to have the *full range* of human emotions, I became alive.

Until that moment, my entire life had been like Pinocchio, a wooden puppet and a slave to doing the right thing. Not only was I a slave to doing the right things, but also to having the "right" thoughts and even feeling the "right" feelings. In therapy, as I learned to allow myself to feel anger, hate, rage, disappointment, jealousy, loneliness, sadness, triumph, success, victory—the *full range* of human emotions—I experienced an enlightened

---

[1] *One of the most powerful lessons I learned in therapy is that there is no such thing as "bad" feelings. Feelings and emotions are neither good nor bad, they simply "are." I will use the term "bad" as a shortcut for painful, shameful, uncomfortable emotions such as guilt, rage, lust, anger, or grief, etc.*

sense of aliveness. I had not previously afforded myself that right. I became a real human being.

To summarize:

> Step 1:
>
> The "Ah" moment is when you discover an emotion you did not know you had. Or, you discover a new depth of that emotion. For example, you may have been aware of annoyance or even anger, but you discover *rage*. Let's call this the discovery of a *primary* hidden emotion. Unearthing this provides emotional relief because a repressed emotion that was there, but unfelt, is now acknowledged. The "Iceberg Analogy of the Human Psyche" diagram at the end of this chapter illustrates the idea of emotions hidden in the unconscious.
>
> Step 2:
>
> However, pain often remains because there is another, *secondary*, hidden thought connected to that primary emotion. That thought is, "It's *wrong* for me to have that (primary) emotion." Recognizing, acknowledging, confronting and validating the secondary emotion is the "Ha" moment that eliminates the need for the pain. That is, when it's OK to have the full range of emotions, then the pain, whose purpose was to protect you from supposedly intolerable emotions, no longer has a purpose and disappears.

THE AHA MOMENT

In my life, discovering that "I have rage towards my father" was the first step. However, feeling that "it's *wrong* for me to have rage towards my father" kept me in pain. The pain distracted me from feeling these painful, shameful, guilty emotions. In treatment, when I finally integrated that it was not only OK, but universal and inevitable to have these types of "bad" feelings, the pain ceased to have a function and went away. To be clear, the healing process does not require the "bad feeling" (in my case, rage towards my father) to disappear, only to be acknowledged and validated. Recognizing, acknowledging, confronting and accepting our emotions ends the need to distract our attention from them and therefore eliminates the need for pain.

Summing up, the combination of uncovering, confronting and accepting suppressed emotions and the hidden "emotion about the emotions," leads to the relief of psychosomatic pain—"Ah-Ha!"

Chapter Addendum

I offer the following thoughts as an addendum to this chapter because the ideas below may not be critical to the relief of physical pain. However, the emotional foundation that has been laid up to this point now opens up unique opportunities for broader healing.

Clearly, I could end my analysis here justified in a conclusion that my dad was over-protective, unsupportive, and unavailable. Acknowledging that these feelings exist, and that it's normal and universal to have them, may likely be enough to eliminate inner conflict and, therefore, pain.

However, it would leave me without much of a relationship with my father. Actually, I would have a relationship with him—it would be difficult, conflicted and tainted with anger and resentment. Interestingly, I have met many people whose parents were highly supportive, encouraging and involved in their activities, only to learn that they were angry and resentful at their parents for being "too involved" and/or for "pressuring" them to perform and excel. So, which is the more true: that dad was over protective, controlling and an emotional threat, or that dad was a powerful role model, a man of integrity, honor and loyalty, whose family and their well-being was his one and only concern? In the world of emotions *both* co-exist and must be validated. In reality, neither view is more true, more valid, or better. Choosing, and articulating one view need not, and must not, invalidate the other. However, embracing one view or the other will produce two very different relationships with my father.

As I become aware of and accept the wide range of my own emotions and humanity, including the extraordinary aspects of my character as well as my flaws and foibles, I have a greater capacity to appreciate the full range of emotions and humanity in others—including my father. I can now feel and express love, compassion, connection, and my deep appreciation for him. Before, I was unable to reconcile the "good" and "bad" emotions I had towards my father and I therefore limited his participation in my life across-the-board. Now, for the most part, I can sort out, separate and acknowledge my emotions. When I feel anger and rage, I can act responsibly. I can also feel and express the love, appreciation, honor and respect that I have and always had for my father. We are now closer than ever. He is a stand for my greatness and a source of strength. Among the countless gifts I received from him, I inherited his powerful psychological aptitude that enabled me to get better, expand our relationship, and be of service to others.

ICEBERG ANALOGY OF THE HUMAN PSYCHE

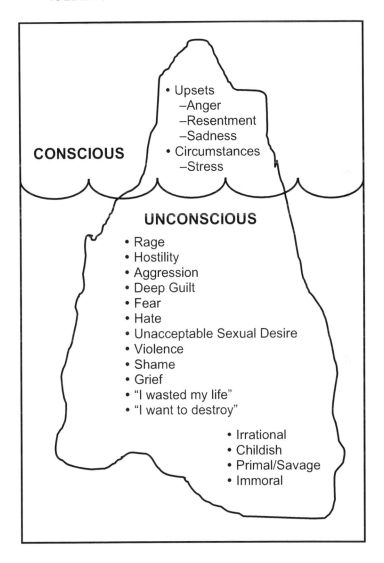

THE AHA MOMENT

NINE

HELPING OTHERS GET BETTER FASTER – CREATION OF THE "ALUMNI PANEL"

For years, my morning routine had become habitually painful. I would awake, pull off the sheets, place my feet on the floor and, as I gingerly applied weight, the pain would shoot up from my second to last left toe, rise past the outer tendon behind my knee, go up around and through my left buttock and zero in on my lower back, just above my waist. Then one morning, as suddenly as it appeared, the pain ceased to exist. While there was still a series of setbacks and breakthroughs yet to come, the war was won.

Several years later, after being pain-free for about three years, I created the "Dr. Sarno Panel Discussion." Each month this panel would feature a line-up of four former patients who went through treatment with Dr. Sarno and became pain-free, each telling their stories about recovery from psychosomatic pain and answering questions from an audience made up of Dr. Sarno's current patients. My intention was that, by interacting with a variety of panelists who had been through the process, patients would get better sooner.

I also envisioned that the panel would be self-perpetuating in the sense that people in the audience who were inspired to do so would eventually appear on the panel when they got better. Dr. Sarno was open to the idea and for over five years and more than 60 monthly panel discussions, the "Alumni Panel," as Dr. Sarno named it in reference to people who have "graduated" from treatment, played an important part in his treatment program for over 5,000 participants.

PART II

APPLYING MINDBODY MEDICINE

The day science begins to study the non-physical phenomena, it will make more progress in one decade than in all the previous centuries of its existence.

—NIKOLA TESLA
U.S. physicist, engineer, and inventor
Born in Croatia (1856–1943)

TEN

QUESTIONS AND ANSWERS

Introduction to Questions and Answers

The following questions and answers are typical of interactions that took place during the Alumni Panel discussions. It is important to remind you that these answers represent my personal experience. They are not prescriptions or medical advice. You will notice that the questions directed to the panelists are in the realm of "What was it like for you?" which only a patient can answer, rather than, "What should I do to get better?" which only a doctor should answer.

QUESTIONS AND ANSWERS

Q: Are you saying that this psychosomatic pain is "all in my head" and that I am not really feeling pain?

A: No. The psychosomatic pain is real and, in fact, "one of the most painful symptoms in medicine."[21] However, the *source* of the pain is not physical, it is psychological. This pain is created by your mind to distract your attention from painful/shameful emotions that it fears are unbearable. The pain starts when a part of your mind detects that unbearable or dangerous feelings currently repressed, or unconscious, may soon become conscious.

Q: What was the source of your pain?

A: This has two answers. Physiologically, the pain occurred when my brain chose to send less oxygen to a particular part of my body. Psychologically, I used that pain to distract my attention from unconscious painful emotions for fear that if I became aware of them it would be unbearable for me and that I may act from these emotions and hurt people I love.

Q: How do I know if the source of my pain is psychosomatic or physical?

A: Only a doctor can make this determination. "No one should assume his or her symptoms are psychologically caused until a physician has ruled out the possibility of a serious disease such as cancer, tumors, bone disease and many other conditions."[22]

Q: Have you ever had back pain again or other symptoms, and how do you deal with them?

A: Yes, over the more than ten years since recovering from back pain, I have had all kinds of symptoms, including short episodes of back pain, diarrhea, sleeplessness, and sharp pains in my feet and shoulders. Without fail, with each of these pains, my first inclination was to look at it from a physical perspective: "My foot is suddenly hurting me—I must have stepped on something wrong" or "Did I sleep with the air conditioner blowing on my neck? It's really sore" or "Did I eat something bad?" Over time, I have become quicker at acknowledging these initial thoughts, and saying to myself, "Wait a second, what's *really* going on? What's going on *emotionally?*"

I'll really get "in there" and "go deep" with myself. I will start to examine my experience psychologically. I'll start to wonder, for example, "Where am I being harsh with myself? I will look at my life and ask, "Where am I making up stories about how I *should* feel or what my life *should* look like?" For example, I might begin to see that I have thoughts such as, "I should be able to deal with this issue easily; my bank account should have more money in it; I should be married by now, or my home should be bigger. As I continue to explore the interior terrain, sometimes the thoughts that turn up get a little nastier, like, "What kind of loser, and miserable failure am I?" I might ask myself, for example, "What did my girlfriend say that hurt my feelings or triggered old self doubts within me? What happened at work? How did I feel about myself when the Amex bill arrived and I didn't have the funds?" Looking at these thoughts on my own is often enough to eliminate the pain. Other times I'll share these thoughts with Dr. Sarno, my therapist, or a trusted friend.

A remarkable trend is also emerging now that almost everyone in my life knows about my experience with mindbody pain. I recently went to work with back soreness, thinking that this time I really did injure my back—probably in yoga class. I sheepishly acknowledged that yes, the author of a book on back pain had a back ache and, after laughing, they said, "don't worry— it's probably nerves about your promotion and the big new project you'll be in charge of. Don't worry you'll be fine." The pain disappeared a few days later.

Please note, if I twist my ankle playing baseball I don't think emotionally, I put ice on it.

Q: Did you have to resolve your life circumstances or change your personality to get rid of your pain?

A: I did not have to resolve my life circumstances or change my personality to eliminate the pain because they were not causing the pain. Clearly, certain life circumstances produce uncomfortable feelings and unconscious conflict between one part of the mind that wants to express these emotions and another part of the mind that feels it would be in the best interests of its owner to *keep* these emotions in the unconscious. Similarly, certain personality traits, such as being good or perfect, compound one's need to relegate "unacceptable" to the unconscious. Pain takes one's attention away from these emotions.

While awareness that circumstances and personality traits play a role in the pain process is important, the critical point is that the presence of pain in mindbody syndromes always signifies the existence of repressed feelings, such as anger and anxiety. Healing does not require changing your circumstances or your personality, or even eliminating these "undesirable" feelings. Healing comes from learning that there is nothing wrong with or inherently dangerous about having these feelings.

Q: Did you need to eliminate unconscious repressed emotions to stop the pain?

A: No, I needed to resolve the conflict I had *about* having these emotions. Conceptually, this involves first acknowledging that these unconscious "bad" emotions actually *exist* in the first place, and second, realizing that it's OK to have them. None of this means that they need to go away or even be expressed.

What this looks like in my life is that while dealing with life circumstances and situations as responsibly and appropriately as I can, I remind myself that it's not the situation that is causing any pain, but it is my *internal reaction* to the situation that is causing pain. For example, my 85-year old father has not changed. He will *still* say things to my sisters, my mother, or me that enrage me. I'll want to scream and yell at him and I can sometimes even feel a primal or savage impulse to want to physically hurt him. I'll think to myself, "I can't believe what he just said. He is such a *bleep!* Do I hit him or call him a name? Of course not! But, I *do* have the thoughts and I now know that it's OK for me to have these thoughts. Before therapy, I was afraid that if I had these types of thoughts, then I would act on them. Therefore my brain deemed these feelings dangerous and found a way to repress them or distract me from them, thereby protecting others and me. (Ironically, the true danger of "acting out" emotions stems from *not* acknowledging them.)

Now that "bad" feelings are no longer "off-limits" or "unthinkable," there is no reason for pain. At times, I may choose to say or do something about a situation, but I have the ability to modulate and be responsible about what I say. I no longer feel like a piece of shit for having shitty feelings. I feel the rage and the anger, and I can even feel primal or childish impulses, but I don't feel like I'm a bad person or a bad son for having those feelings. I don't think that there is anything wrong with me, or that it's bad or *wrong* for me to have those feelings and therefore I do not experience pain. In life, there will always be difficult circumstances and even painfully devastating situations that need to be dealt with and some that *can't* be changed. Now, thanks to this education and newfound knowledge, I can deal with them pain-free.

Q: Do life circumstances still produce rage in you?

A: Of course life circumstances produce rage in me! Sometimes I express my rage and sometimes I don't, but generally I am aware of it. I'm getting better at minimizing the unconscious conflict I previously described. As a result, I experience little psychosomatic pain. When I'm dealing with difficult life circumstances, I remind myself to be gentle, kind, compassionate, and understanding with myself. I try to deal with that angry, hurt, frightened, or ashamed part of me that judges itself as insufficient, inadequate, and incompetent, as if that part of me were a child. Dr. Sarno reminds us that "a parent, an adult, and a child reside inside our brains and... they are often at odds with one another."[23]

Q: Why do I still feel pain if I can, and do, freely express my rage and anger?

A. I discovered that the rage and anger I expressed in fights or arguments was not what was causing the pain. Dr. Sarno is clear that it is the *unconscious* emotions that are the cause of psychosomatic pain.[24] Therefore, the pain is connected to feelings *other* than what a person is yelling about. The screaming becomes another sideshow, in addition to the pain, to distract the yeller from painful emotions. In other words, the screaming and ensuing drama is yet another distraction designed to keep the screamer from looking at his or her "hidden" emotions.

I once met a young mother with psychosomatic pain who shared with me that she yelled at her children all the time. She read Dr. Sarno's books and was obviously aware of her anger towards her children, and could not understand why she still had pain. She shared with me that in therapy, she discovered that what she had not been willing to confront, and therefore needed to suppress and "distract herself from" were feelings of insufficiency as a mother, resentment towards her children for limiting her freedom, and an irrational wish (from time to time) that her children not exist at all. Clearly, prior to confronting and accepting these emotions, her mind needed to insure that these emotions were not felt, and used pain as a distraction. When she discovered and accepted this, her pain disappeared. Healing comes, not from the absence of such emotions, but from the understanding that such emotions are "normal" and "universal." She realized that the existence of such emotions does not mean she is a horrible mother or that she would act on her emotions.

It is also noteworthy that many people get better immediately just by reading Dr. Sarno's books—without doing deep psychological work or profound self inquiry. How I envy these people! They simply accept that (1) there is nothing physically wrong with them, and (2) that their pain is there to distract their attention from painful, unconscious emotions. Period. They have seen the tip of their emotional iceberg and have no need to go on a scuba diving expedition in icy, shark infested waters to believe that there is mass of unconscious rage below the surface. They get it. Good for them. May you be one of

QUESTIONS AND ANSWERS

these fortunate folks and may this book accelerate your progress.

Q: I'm doing everything Dr. Sarno's says to do, but I still feel pain. What would you do?

A: Dr. Sarno points out that, the occurrence of psychosomatic pain *always* signifies the presence of painful/dangerous unconscious feelings that are threatening to become conscious.[25]

There was a time in my treatment when I was working hard at looking at my personality and emotions, reflecting on my past, and thinking about my life circumstances, but still had pain. What I needed to confront was that I was still *not OK* with having certain emotions. The pain served to distract my attention from what my mind perceived to be dangerous, shameful, guilt-ridden, or otherwise unacceptable emotions. Pain indicated that my emotional search needed to go wider or deeper. By wider, I mean uncovering more areas, or sources, of unacceptable emotions from my childhood, personality, or circumstances. By deeper, I mean examining the magnitude of these emotions and my *reactions to* them. In my case, I still had pain because while I was willing to accept that I was angry at my father, I was not yet willing to accept that I had *rage* towards my father because that would mean that I was an unloving and ungrateful son.

Psychosomatic treatment requires a patient's psychological effort. You can use your typical "Dr. Sarno patient" personality traits, such as being a hard-working, thorough, meticulous, and driven perfectionist, to your advantage. Bring your diligence to the task at hand. It really takes work to retrain your mind away from over-learned habits and automatic, painful, "Pavlovian" responses to suppressed emotions. Instead of directing your attention and diligence outwardly towards the physical realm, like I did at first by researching the biomechanics of back pain, visiting countless doctors, and pursuing physical remedies, you could direct that inquiry inwardly.

The physical inquiry plays right into the hand of the psychosomatic syndrome by distracting your attention from painful emotions. When you are able to look at the thoughts you were afraid to look at, the symptoms no longer serve a purpose and disappear. Do whatever works for you: journaling, writing, therapy, or speaking with the right friends. Asking for help is a particularly novel, unfamiliar, and effective approach and remedy for typical mindbody sufferers who often think they can do it all on their own.

QUESTIONS AND ANSWERS

Q: What was one of the most challenging aspects of the healing process?

A: One of the most difficult challenges was to deal with the *doubt* of the diagnosis, or my "skepticism." A quote often attributed to Mark Twain comes to mind: "It ain't so much the things we don't know that get us into trouble. It's the things we know that just ain't so." The doubt is difficult to deal with because there is strong agreement within society that the source of pain is physical. Worse, it has become more than agreement, it has become common knowledge. The popular understanding is that if you have chronic, debilitating back pain, then you certainly have a physical problem that may even require surgery. The fact that almost everyone "knows" that a herniated disk leads to pain points to the widespread and necessarily epidemic proportions of the syndrome. I say, "necessarily epidemic" because psychosomatic pain does not come knocking at your door saying, *"Hi, I'm just psychosomatic. Don't worry about me. There really isn't anything physically wrong with you."* It comes at you with the most believable, plausible, and socially and personally acceptable disguise it can create, so as to *demand* your attention.

At this point in history, one of the most believable disguises for psychosomatic symptoms is back pain. It may even come with evidence. Even the MRI is telling you it's physical. As an engineer, I could read the MRI and see the disk bulge next to the sciatic nerve. When I read the MRI and understood it, I was trapped. I had many doctors, in crisp white lab coats, impressive offices, and state-of-the-art hospitals who were written up as the best doctors in New York tell me I needed surgery. *That* creates doubt. So, how do you deal with that? How do you deal with having doubt, day-in and day-out, and still pursue the mental approach to your own healing?

You begin by accepting that doubt is part of the process. You don't wait for the doubt to go away. If I asked you if you wanted to get better, you would say, "Yes, of course." But, the truth is, a part of you *doesn't* want to get better. That's the part that wants your suppressed emotions to *stay* suppressed; the part that thinks it's doing you a favor, protecting you and others. That's the part of you that's going to create doubt. The doubt is one more powerful distraction designed to keep you from looking at your emotions.

In my case, a part of my mind didn't want me to go anywhere near the rage I felt towards my father and how I would feel about myself if I were to become aware of that rage. A part of me was afraid of what I might say or do to my father. In therapy, I gained emotional maturity, or, you can say, I acquired emotional education. I learned that just having certain emotions doesn't make me a bad person. I learned that just because I feel something doesn't mean I will automatically act out of that feeling. Before I learned this, it was necessary for me to suppress my emotions and therefore doubt the diagnosis. Doubt is normal. If you didn't doubt, you wouldn't have pain! Paradoxically, on one hand, you have to give up the doubt to get better. On the other hand, doubt is an inevitable part of the process. *Be willing* to give up the doubt.

Q: What else can I do to deal with my skepticism?

A: You are doing it. By reading this book you are gaining knowledge and knowledge is the remedy. Seek out and speak with patients who have become pain free. People who get better, love to support and empower others. Check out the web and book resources in the back of this book. When you get better, help someone else get better. That *really* eliminates doubt.

Q: Dr. Sarno says symptoms are designed to be distractions from unconscious rage.[26] How do you deal with unconscious emotions if they are unconscious?

A: The key is to make the *connection* between one's unconscious emotions and one's pain. How much of that repressed emotion needs to become conscious in order for someone to make that connection is up to the individual. Some people don't need to see much evidence in order to make the connection between their unconscious emotions and their pain. That's why thousands of people have gotten better just by reading Dr. Sarno's books and, my intention is that many more will by reading this book. They may not need to confront specific painful/shameful emotions to *acknowledge* that they are there and are the source of the pain. Some of us do need to begin to feel them in order to acknowledge their presence. For those of us, we eventually learn that there is nothing to fear in confronting painful/shameful emotions. You won't die. You won't kill anyone. They're just emotions. It's normal to have a full range of emotions. Every human being has a full range of emotions, even though many of us do not allow ourselves to feel most of them. As you accept and acknowledge your emotions, you can have emotions, and they won't have you.

THE NATURE OF THE RELATIONSHIP BETWEEN PAIN AND EMOTIONS

The next three questions are designed to address the nature of the relationship between *psychosomatic pain and unconscious emotions*. This is essential to understand because the relationship establishes the remedy. The particular correlation between pain and emotions

QUESTIONS AND ANSWERS

distinguished below explains why patients get better simply by understanding the nature of the psychosomatic process and why the corresponding emotional therapeutic process has produced consistent results in thousands of cases.

Q: I am willing to accept that I have repressed emotions I do not want to feel. Do you mean that the physical pain is a way of my body expressing emotional pain?

A: No. The relationship between the pain and the emotions where the pain is a kind of "physical expression" of the repressed emotions is <u>not</u> what is causing your pain.

The "pain as physical expression of unconscious emotions" model does not explain why patients get better just by learning that the mere existence of unbearable unconscious emotions are at the root of the pain. These people have not changed their circumstances or lessened the extent of their emotional pain, yet the pain ceases.

If physical pain was the expression of emotional pain, you would have to eliminate, or at least reduce the magnitude of, repressed emotions that are theoretically trying to express themselves through pain. This would be very difficult to do because you can't consciously express unconscious emotions, and also because they are continuously being replenished.

This explains why I never experienced any pain relief from the numerous occasions I screamed at my father at the top of my lungs giving him a "piece of my mind." This never provided any physical relief, because I was expressing *conscious* rage, or emotions I was aware of. Expressing my anger, often does not address the underlying conflicts such as "I *shouldn't* be angry at my father" and "I'm angry at myself." Therefore, no matter how much I yelled and screamed, the pain persisted.

I've heard of emotional relief processes where you yell in the woods or punch pillows. I believe this is useful to verify the vast amounts of rage stockpiled in the unconscious. However, without, a visceral understanding that these emotions are normal and universal, they will continue to be threatening and cause pain.

Q: Are you saying that I am experiencing symptoms because I may be getting some kind of indirect benefit from having pain?

A: No. This "Secondary Gain" theory, which asserts that people have pain in order to avoid doing things they don't want to do, or get things that they do want such as attention or affection, is not what is causing your pain.

The problem with this theory is that it still requires a physical explanation for pain and does not explain why people get better from simply acknowledging that unconscious emotions are at the root of the pain.

QUESTIONS AND ANSWERS

This theory also runs counter to my personal observation of hundreds of mindbody patients (including myself) who do exactly the opposite of shirking responsibility or getting a reward. We find a way to work, travel, care-take parents, and raise children—even *with* excruciating pain. We are so driven that we will push ourselves to accomplish tasks even if it means having a cot in the office, attending meetings while lying down, flying on airplanes standing up, limping from one doctor appointment to another, using an infinite assortment of heat packs, ice packs, braces, belts, cushions, and endless amounts of pain medication.

Q: What *is* the relationship between pain and unconscious emotions?

A: Psychosomatic pain exists to *distract your attention* away from unconscious emotions such as rage, anger, shame or sadness. A part of your mind thinks it would be unbearable, intolerable and dangerous for you to become consciously aware of these feelings. When your "unconscious reservoir" is full and threatens to boil over and spill out into consciousness, a pain/distraction mechanism is induced by the brain, utilizing something that would demand your attention twenty-four hours a day, seven days a week so that you would *never* focus on these "dangerous" emotions. Your brain thinks it is doing you a favor, or protecting you, by insuring that these emotions remain hidden from your consciousness.

Relief comes not from eliminating these unconscious emotions, but by eliminating their threat. This clearly explains why when you learn that it is normal and universal to have such feelings, the pain ceases to serve a function and disappears.

In my life, once I accepted that I had both love *and* rage towards my father and that this was not only OK, but universal, or part and parcel of being human, the pain disappeared.

More Questions and Answers

Q: Are you suggesting that I may be inflicting this horrible pain on myself? I am beginning to feel outraged, insulted and offended. I have medical evidence that indicates the source of my pain is physical.

A: Yes, I am. I understand that this is a bitter, jagged pill to swallow, but if you are willing to accept that you are doing this, then you may stop. Remember that psychosomatic pain is created by your mind to distract your attention from painful/shameful emotions that it fears are unbearable. The pain starts when a part of your mind detects that these unbearable or dangerous feelings that are currently repressed, or unconscious, may soon become conscious. The mind is powerfully guarded against these feelings ever seeing the light of day, lest the humiliating and horrific "truth" about you be exposed. At best the mind is deceptive, and at worst, vehemently hostile in its defense efforts (hence, your outrage). Your brain thinks it is protecting you. The cost is terrible pain. Healing comes from learning that what I have been hiding is harmless, benign and not only commonplace, but universally human. When the pain no longer serves a function (to prevent the emergence or protect you from what it perceives to be painful/shameful/dangerous emotions) it disappears.

Q: If I accept that the source of my pain is emotional and not physical, does that mean that I am defective, or weak in some way?

A: I confronted this when I chose to begin psychotherapy. For years I secretly wanted to see a psychotherapist, but I did not think it was manly and I also thought that I should be able to solve my own problems. Going to therapy, I feared, would be an admission that there was something mentally wrong with me. Now, with the excuse that this was for "my back," I justified going to therapy. In therapy, not only did I heal my back pain, every area of my life benefitted. I discovered the world of emotions. I realized that I had been limiting my emotional life to a very narrow band of feelings that were not too "bad" and not too "good." In therapy, I gained access to the full spectrum of human emotions. I also peeked into the world of the unconscious and saw its dramatic impact on my emotional and physical well being. While I discovered there was nothing wrong with me, there was certainly a world of emotional knowledge and education that I was missing. With the guidance of Dr. Eric Sherman, my therapist, I looked at enough emotional iceberg tips to know that there was vastly more "beneath the surface."

A great and wise friend of mine, Jeffrey Mironov, says, "The human mind is a seething and brooding cauldron of discontent and denial, simmering with anguish, guilt, shame, and rage of barbaric and savage proportions threatening to boil over at any moment." Not only does this align with Dr. Sarno's model and explain why it seems imperative that these "bad" feelings not be permitted to spill out into our consciousness, Jeffrey's statement also points directly to the universality of this condition. Dr. Sarno says, "Psychosomatic phenomena are not a form of illness. They must be seen as part of the human condition—to which everyone is susceptible."[27] It takes great courage to face, confront *and be responsible* for what lies in our unconscious. The extent to which we can "own" this part of our mind is the extent to which we will not unconsciously "act out," or need to distract ourselves from these emotions.

QUESTIONS AND ANSWERS

The overwhelming majority of people are unwilling to "face their demons." To this end, Dr. Sarno estimates that, "in the United States only 10 to 20 percent of people with psychosomatic disorders are able to accept the fact that their symptoms are emotional in origin. Many are downright hostile to the idea."[28] Most of us prefer to live in a world of blame, accusation and victimization. Most of us *want* the cause of the pain to be physical so that it can be cut out of us or medicated, so as not to have to confront that "seething cauldron of discontent." I think everyone should be trained in the ways of the mind and in the dynamics of feelings and emotions. If all politicians, CEOs, teachers, clergy and indeed, all people who are responsible for other people did some form of psychotherapy, therapy or mind training, the world would look very different.

Q: What is meant by "location substitution" and "symptom imperative?"

A: If the symptoms of your pain condition are removed without addressing the true cause of your pain (distraction from unwanted unconscious emotions) then your mind will find it imperative, or necessary, to produce another distraction. This is often accomplished by changing the location of the pain to another area of your body or simply waiting it out and having the pain return to the same place, depending on what would be most credible to you. In addition, based on my conversations with many chronic pain sufferers, I have also noticed that the mind will gladly settle for new "non-physical" distractions such as a messy divorce, romantic fixation or work obsession.

In my recovery process the "symptom imperative" process happened twice. The first time was prior to my introduction to mindbody medicine when I had cortisone steroids injected into my lower back. I was so convinced that this procedure would work, that it did. It removed the symptoms, by way of the placebo effect (*the beneficial effect in a patient following a particular treatment that arises from the patient's expectations concerning the treatment rather than from the treatment itself.*[29]) Since the emotional root cause of the pain had not been addressed, the pain returned, in this case to the same exact place.

In the later stages of my recovery, after considerable work with my psychotherapist, when the sciatica that once raced down my left leg began to fade away, I started to experience pain down my *other* leg. At first, I thought that the herniation must have moved. But after applying rigorous thought and remembering the herniation had been on my right side for years, the idea that it would suddenly move, or bulge out into another direction became laughable and the pain disappeared. Then, a few days later, I started to experience pain in my right shoulder. This initially scared me, so I discussed it with my therapist. It became clear to me that this was such an obvious case of "location substitution" that, after years of being convinced that I had a structural abnormality, the "jig was up." I finally exposed my mind's emotional trickery and had the "pain on the run." Within days the pain disappeared once and for all.

Q: What can I do to get better?

A: Inevitably, someone would always ask this question at the panel discussions and we would immediately hear Dr. Sarno vociferously clear his throat, reminding the panelists that while we could talk about our personal experiences, only a qualified medical professional could give treatment advice. I will therefore summarize Dr. Sarno's recommended treatment plan and share with you, as I have done throughout the book, what I did to get better.

In the beginning of Chapter 4 of *The Divided Mind*, titled "Treatment," Dr. Sarno says, "What you need to get better... is not a leap of faith but a leap of understanding." I hope this book has deepened your understanding of Dr. Sarno's principles and that you have begun the necessary next phase of infusing this knowledge into your psyche, so as to be able to act on this knowledge and change your brain's old response mechanisms. We *can* influence our unconscious, automatic thought patterns by the conscious application of mind. We can end old habitual ways of thinking and create new ones. As I have previously stated, the cure rests not only in more information, but also in being able to think differently.

It's important to keep in mind that since there isn't anything structurally wrong with your body, nothing damaged, nothing broken, the amount of time that you have been in pain is not an indication of how much time it will take you to recover. You should not even be concerned if you have had numerous recurrent pain episodes since the start of your symptoms.

The two foundational building blocks upon which Dr. Sarno's therapeutic program rests are:

Repudiate the Physical – Say to yourself that "there is nothing wrong with my body" (assuming you have had a consultation with a qualified physician). Any structural abnormalities that have been found on an X-ray or MRI are normal changes associated with age.[30]

Accept the Psychological – Your pain is due to a harmless condition, initiated by the brain to serve a psychological purpose. There's nothing psychologically wrong with you, either. You are not "weak" or mentally deficient, defective or ill. This physiologic reaction to unconscious thoughts is normal and universal to all human beings.[31]

QUESTIONS AND ANSWERS

THE DAILY REMINDERS

In *Healing Back Pain*, Dr. Sarno recommends a daily review of what he calls the "Daily Reminders." "Patients are given a list of twelve key thoughts, and it is suggested that at least once a day they set aside fifteen minutes or so when they can relax and quietly review them."[32]

- The pain is due to TMS, not to structural abnormalities
- The direct reason for the pain is mild oxygen deprivation
- TMS is a harmless condition, caused by my repressed emotions
- The principle emotion is my repressed anger
- TMS exists only to distract my attention from the emotions
- Since my back is basically normal there is nothing to fear
- Therefore physical activity is not dangerous
- And I must resume all physical activity
- I will not be concerned or intimidated by the pain
- I will shift my attention from the pain to emotional issues
- I intend to be in control – not my subconscious mind

- I must think psychologically at all times, not physically

The Daily Study Program

In *The Divided Mind*, Dr. Sarno outlines the basic steps of the "Daily Study Program"[33] which he gave people who had a consultation with him and attended his basic lectures.

Read and continue re-reading the book or books you are using a bit at a time. I recommend you set a specific "dosage" for yourself such as 10 pages a day or 20 minutes a day. I recommend using a highlighter or underlining passages that jump out at you or remind you of yourself.

Set aside time every day to perform this work.

Remind yourself that *unconscious* feelings are at the source of your pain, not conscious feelings or stress, such as being angry with your boss, kids, parents, etc.

Make a list of the *conscious* feelings, thoughts or circumstances that may be contributing to the unconscious feelings.

Write an essay about each item on your list. For each item on your list examine the following factors that may contribute to the internal reservoir of rage, rendering it

QUESTIONS AND ANSWERS

on the brink of capacity and on the verge of spilling over into consciousness:

- **Childhood experiences**, such as excessive discipline, neglect, abuse, expectations, leave large amount of pain, sadness, guilt, regret and anger in the unconscious.

- **Personality traits** make the "greatest contribution" to the internal emotional pain and anger. "If you drive yourself to be perfect, to achieve, to succeed, if you are your own severest critic, if you are very conscientious, these are likely to make you very angry inside."

- **Life Pressures and circumstances** also contribute to internal rage.

- Consider that **mortality** (your own and others') is a source of rage that is very difficult to be consciously aware of, as is anger within a **close personal relationship** such as a parent, spouse or child.

Add any situations where you become consciously annoyed or angry but cannot express it.

I have found that meeting with other people who are well versed in the mindbody medicine principles put forth in this book can be helpful. Be aware of the pitfalls of comparing yourself to others who seem to be getting better faster, leaving you wishing you were one of them, or, comparing yourself to others who seem to be making little or no progress, leaving you afraid of being one of them.

Additionally, about 20 percent of patients who worked with Dr. Sarno also worked with one of his psychologists to complete the process. I was one of them and this wonderful work not only eliminated my pain, but I've also benefited in every area of my life from being more aware of the workings of my mind.

A practice that worked very effectively for me was to do my journaling immediately following my therapy sessions. I used what we discussed as points of departure that would inevitably lead to a rich exploration of uncharted internal terrain.

The Treasure Map Process

A process that I developed that works for me to this day for dealing with early signs of pain is what I call *The Treasure Map Process*.

QUESTIONS AND ANSWERS

Step 1. Describe the pain.

Example: My right foot hurts. I feel fine when I am sitting or lying down, but, it hurts every time I put weight on it. It's a sharp pain between the ball of my foot and my heel. It doesn't hurt as much in the morning. It hurts more as the day goes on.

Step 2. Pretend your life is a treasure map. Scan the terrain of your life and identify a situation or circumstance that is upsetting or bothering you. This will be the "X that marks the spot" for where to start "digging down" towards your unconscious in the next steps. Use one situation for Steps 3 -6. Rework the steps for as many other situations as they occur to you.

Example: I'm upset about recently ending a romantic relationship.

Step 3. Describe the facts about what happened or what is happening.

Example: Linda and I were together for two years. Last week she told me that in this coming year she wants to move back home to England, and that she would like me to go with her and start a family. She had mentioned this a year ago and I told her I needed time to think about it. When I told her last week that I did not want to move to England at this time, she thanked me for my honesty and chose to end our relationship.

Step 4. Write about your thoughts and feelings about the situation. Feel free to include any related thoughts about yourself or your childhood.

Example: I am so angry at Linda for breaking up with me. I cannot believe she said ___. She should have handled things differently. How could she have done that to me after being together for two years? She is so cold and cruel. What she should have done is ___. I hate her. Why do women always ___? I am so damn frustrated. I am never going to be in a great relationship. Everyone else is in a great relationship. Not one person I know has a great relationship. I am scared of being alone for the rest of my life. Who will take care of me when I'm old? No one outside of my family really cares about me. I am so sad. I feel like a failure. Even mom and dad, who love each other, always fought. Relationships suck. Why can't I ever make one work? I'm not sure if I want to have kids. I don't think I could afford to have kids. Having kids would be so wonderful and fulfilling. They would care about me. Having kids would dominate my life and take away my freedom.

Step 5. Write about the thoughts and feelings you have <u>about</u> your thoughts and feelings in Step 4.

Example: Linda loved me and I should not be angry at her. She loved me and I let her walk away, I'm so ungrateful. She's probably already with someone else. I'm such a loser. I'm not sure I wanted to stay together with her myself, therefore I don't have a right to feel sad, lonely, afraid or angry. I feel guilty. I'm *ashamed of being single at this stage of my life. I should have been able to commit to her. What's wrong with me? I'm such a wimp. I'm so mean. At this point in my life, I should know if I want kids or not. Since I can't afford to have children and buy a house, I must have wasted my Columbia University degree. I've already thrown away my professional career. I think I wasted my life.*

Please note that in Step 5, it is important to remember that you are not attempting to uncover the full depths of the human unconscious mind. You are uncovering enough of the tip of the iceberg to acknowledge a huge mass of unconscious grievances below the surface. You will never be fully aware of your unconscious. At the deeper levels of your unconsciousness you may find self inflicted disappointment, shame, anger, rage and emotional cruelty.

Step 6. Acknowledge that your thoughts and feelings (in Steps 5 and 6) are just thoughts and feelings. Their existence does not mean that you are a bad person for having them, or that it is wrong to have these feelings or that you should be ashamed of having these feelings. Have compassion for yourself and your humanness. You can call this forgiveness, acceptance, self-love, or any other expression that resonates or appeals to you. While Step 6 is mostly an internal shift in perception, you may notice new thoughts and feelings. If so, write them down.

Example: I love, respect, honor, and accept myself just the way I am. I did the best I could and am doing the best I can and that is enough. I am enough. There is nothing wrong with me for having "bad" feelings. I am loving and lovable. I honor and accept Linda's choice. Linda did and is doing the best she can. Though we are not together I wish her well. I appreciate my life and the people who are in it. They are the people who have made me who I am today.

Step 6 is not the disappearance of any feelings or a change in the circumstances. Step 6 is an acknowledgement and acceptance of your feelings as a normal, universal and an inevitable aspect of being human.

Furthermore, the forgiveness I refer to is for giving yourself the "room" or "space" to experience the full range of human emotions, even if they are illogical, mean, selfish, childish, brutal, hurtful, vengeful, or spiteful. It is not necessary to act upon these feelings, or to voice or share these feelings with the other person(s) involved or anyone else, although you may choose to do so. There may be actions to take, conversations to have, and things to work out, but it need not involve physical pain. The key is forgiving oneself and no one can do this for you. Even if others forgive you, unless you forgive

QUESTIONS AND ANSWERS

yourself there will still be unbearable unconscious conflict and resulting pain.

The Treasure Map Process – Worksheets

Here is a worksheet for you to apply *The Treasure Map Process*. I strongly recommend writing it out, and using a clean page for each step. While Steps 4 and 5 are distinct, there certainly is an overlap here, so do not be concerned about getting it right.

Step 1. Describe the pain.

_____
_____
_____
_____
_____
_____
_____
_____
_____
_____
_____
_____

USE YOUR MIND TO HEAL YOUR BODY

Step 2. Identify a situation or circumstance that is upsetting you or bothering you.

QUESTIONS AND ANSWERS

Step 3. Describe the facts about what happened or what is happening.

_____
_____
_____
_____
_____
_____
_____
_____
_____
_____
_____
_____
_____
_____
_____
_____
_____
_____
_____
_____
_____
_____
_____
_____

Step 4. Write about your thoughts and feelings about the situation. Feel free to include any related thoughts about your personality and your childhood.

QUESTIONS AND ANSWERS

Step 5. Write about the thoughts and feelings you have <u>about</u> your thoughts and feelings in Step 4.

Step 6. Acknowledge that your thoughts and feelings (in Steps 5 and 6) are just thoughts and feelings. Their existence does not mean that you are a bad person for having them, or that it is wrong to have these feelings, or that you should be ashamed of having these feelings. Have compassion for yourself and your humanness. You can call this forgiveness, acceptance, self-love, or any expression that resonates or appeals to you.

While Step 6 is mostly an internal shift in perception, you may notice new thoughts and feelings that speak of your innocence or "OK-ness". If so, write them down.

_____
_____
_____
_____
_____
_____
_____
_____
_____
_____
_____
_____

QUESTIONS AND ANSWERS

For a particular pain syndrome, repeat Steps 3-6 for as many situations or circumstances (Step 2) that are upsetting you or bothering you as they come to mind.

Some of you will get better just by reading this book. For those of you who have, you have without doubt accepted there is nothing physically wrong with you, you've realized that your symptoms were there to protect you, by way of distraction from the threat of unconscious emotions rising to your awareness. Congratulations.

For those of you who do not get better right away, this is the part of the book where you will have to go to work. The presence of symptoms simply means that you are still ashamed, afraid or otherwise uncomfortable with certain feelings in your unconscious. The various types and forms of exercises described in this section were designed for you to acknowledge the existence of unconscious emotions so that you can experience firsthand that they are harmless and do not mean anything about you. It is not important that you do these exercises perfectly, what matters is that you do them *every day*, until you get better.

Q: Are you implying that all back surgery is unnecessary?

A: I am not saying that all back surgery is unnecessary. Advancements in spinal surgery, orthopedics and physical therapy have undoubtedly resulted in countless lives being restored to normal. Severe trauma, such as that resulting from falls or automobile accidents clearly must be treated physically. Furthermore, pain syndromes must always be properly examined and tested by a doctor to rule out serious disorders such as cancer, tumors, bone disease and many other conditions.[34] In countless situations, spinal surgeons are life savers.

That being said, in recent years several articles in the *New England Journal of Medicine*, *The Journal of American Medicine*, *The New York Times* and *The New Yorker* have questioned the value of certain types of back surgery and the possible overuse of spine surgery.[35]

Q: Almost every book I've read on the subject of back pain has back exercises. Do they help?

A: While back exercises in and of themselves are not harmful, they imply that a physical condition is causing the pain, draw attention away from a psychological inquiry and are therefore counterproductive.[36] An overall workout that may include back exercises would of course be beneficial to anyone. I do yoga regularly not only for general health benefits but also to vividly reinforce my understanding that there is nothing wrong with my back and that it is healthy and strong.

QUESTIONS AND ANSWERS

Q: I have been working with a psychotherapist for many years. Why do I still have pain?

A: As we have seen, there is a specific relationship between your pain and your symptoms. That is, pain exists to distract attention from painful and unbearable emotions. If your therapist is not aware of this dynamic, you (and your therapist) will likely continue to think that the pain is entirely or partially caused by a physical condition and the pain will persist and continue to successfully perform its function to deter your exploration of painful emotions. This is why I recommend that you work with a medical doctor who is trained to distinguish organically caused pain from psychologically caused pain and, if necessary, a psychotherapist trained in the mind-body connection as described in this book. See "Recommended References" section.

Q: In addition to Dr. Sarno's work, what peer-reviewed medical literature exists regarding the psychosomatic treatment of pain?

A: The medical establishment's historic lack of interest with the psychosomatic treatment of pain disorders "borders on the criminal"[37] according to Dr. Sarno. Despite this unfortunate past, there is rapidly growing attention being given to this subject matter. *The Tension Myositis Syndrome* (TMS) *Wiki*, found online (http://www.tmswiki.org) cites hundreds of articles, books and presentations about the most important research relevant to the psychosomatic treatment of pain published in the world's most reputable and prestigious medical journals such as *The New England Journal of Medicine, International Journal of Epidemiology, Spine, Archives of Physical Medicine and Rehabilitation, British Journal of Psychiatry, Journal of Rheumatology, Journal of the American Medical Association,* and the *New York Times,* to name a few. The TMS *Wiki* summarizes:

1. There is peer-reviewed evidence that adopting TMS [mindbody] techniques can very significantly reduce chronic pain suffering.

2. There is strong peer-reviewed evidence that psychosomatic factors affect perception of pain, development of symptoms and success of surgery.

3. There is peer-reviewed evidence that journaling and meditation can reduce pain in chronic pain sufferers and improve general health.

4. There is strong peer-reviewed evidence that many structural diagnoses of back abnormalities based solely on MRI scans are flawed.

5. There is strong peer-reviewed evidence of the physical symptoms that stress both causes and exacerbates pain in the body.

6. *There is peer-reviewed evidence of the spread of conditions like whiplash in an epidemic-like manner – where it is the preconception of injury which predicts development of the condition.*[38]

Entries from the "Annotated Bibliography" of mindbody research compiled by *The Tension Myositis Syndrome Wiki* researchers can be found under the **Recent Research in the Field of Mindbody Medicine** section included at the end of this book. Please refer to the *Wiki* site for a "Complete Bibliography."

Q: Why has psychosomatic diagnosis and treatment not received more attention and recognition from mainstream medicine?
A: The answer points to the power and threat of psychosomatic medicine. It is powerful in the sense that people trained in mindbody principles discover that they *can* take responsibility for *their own* health and well being. This is why Dr. Sarno never claims to have "healed" or "cured" anyone—patients can only cure themselves. However, this power to heal oneself comes at the cost of acknowledging that "I am doing this to myself." Of course, this idea is threatening and typically sets off feelings of guilt and defensiveness and is subsequently vehemently denied.

USE YOUR MIND TO HEAL YOUR BODY

The idea of people being able to "heal themselves" is also threatening to people who fear they may not be up to the task.

Perhaps most importantly, people do not *want* to confront inner emotions, such as anger, guilt, rage, shame, sadness and fear. Rather than face them, most of us prefer to be "healed" by someone else. We *want* the pain to be something that can be "cut out" or medicated. So, for people who demand to be medicated or have procedures done to them, the medical industry will be all too glad to comply. Sadly, these remedies are largely ineffective, have led to the proliferation of pain syndromes to epidemic proportions, rendering the health care system in a state of crisis, and worst of all left millions of people suffering needlessly.

Clearly, psychosomatic medicine is also threatening to the billion-dollar pain management industry from which countless doctors, pharmaceutical companies, medical device industries, hospitals, and other practitioners profit enormously.

We must confront that this vast supply is in direct proportion to society's demand to have someone or something else "fix them." As with the war on drugs, where victory comes not by stopping the supply but by dealing with the demand, the legitimacy, availability of psychosomatic treatment will come to light when we stop insisting that someone else cure us.

QUESTIONS AND ANSWERS

As a society, we are just beginning to summon the necessary courage and willingness to face our deepest fears of who and what we think we are. On the other side of this inevitable confrontation, however, lies the future of medicine, the knowledge and understanding of our innocence, and true healing.

PART III

YOUR ROLE

Let your mind dance with your body.

—Yogi Tea

ELEVEN

ENDING PAIN FOREVER

By their very nature, psychosomatic disorders require an environment of general public agreement, or consensus, to execute their mission, which is to grab a hold of your attention and not let go. To do so, these disorders must carry a compelling, socially acceptable line of reasoning. Everyone "knows" that their back pains are due to something physical that happened. Is the problem a pull, a strain, a sprain, or heaven forbid, a disk abnormality? If the dreaded disk abnormality is indicated on an MRI, everyone "knows" that surgery is likely. Similarly, everyone "knows" carpal tunnel syndrome is due to over-usage of computer keyboards, and acne is due to clogged pores. The idea that a physical cause to these disorders may not exist is, by and large, unimaginable. The thought that the pain is emotionally induced to serve a psychological purpose is currently inconceivable.

While the healing of one person's symptoms requires information, the eradication of a nationwide mindbody epidemic requires an informational campaign. This movement depends on you.

With today's acceptability level of psychosomatic principles ranging from dismissible and laughable to vehemently attacked, individuals must beat overwhelming odds to overcoming their pain condition—*if* they manage to learn this option even exists. Indeed, merely discovering the mindbody treatment option has become no easy feat. In a move that defies reason, even the American Psychiatric Association has removed the term "psychosomatic" from their official publication, the *Diagnostic and Statistical Manual of Mental Disorders* (DSM). Calling this action "scandalous" and "heinous," Dr. Sarno says "you might as well remove the word infection from medical dictionaries."[39]

The financial incentives of the multi-billion dollar pain management machine are staggering. Common chronic pain conditions run up $560-635 billion annually in direct medical treatment costs and lost productivity.[40] An online search for back pain, or carpel tunnel, fibromyalgia, acne, migraines produce thousands of articles describing the physical cause and cure approach. In the rare instances where a connection between pain and emotions *is* acknowledged, it is marginalized as a contributing factor.

The problem is that conventional physical diagnosis and treatment is simply not working. The result of this miscarriage of medicine is a nationwide pain epidemic that has reached catastrophic proportions. Approximately 100 million U.S. adults—more than the number affected by heart disease, diabetes, and cancer combined—suffer from chronic pain conditions.[41] The false foundation of physically centered solutions to chronic pain is unsustainable over time.

Peer-reviewed articles published in the world's most reputable and prestigious medical journals are beginning to question the effectiveness and incentives of structural procedures and pharmaceutical fixes.

We need to make the psychosomatic diagnosis socially and medically acceptable. It is the privilege of those of us who have overcome this vicious, yet benign, and therefore needless, malady to make it easier for others to heal themselves.

What can you do? **Let others know.** Share your stories, your challenges and your victories. When one person demonstrates the real healing power of accepting emotions that were once perceived as dangerous, other people will have a greater chance to do the same.

The proof of the pudding is in the eating. People who learn about mindbody medicine get better. People in vast numbers will get better through the methods described and referenced in this and similar books. We need to make mindbody medicine water cooler and kitchen conversation. With the advent of social media and the Internet, our ability to share ourselves and what the possibility of mindbody medicine has to offer people is growing exponentially.

Take Action Now! In addition to sharing with your friends, family and colleagues, I have set up a webpage, **UseMindBody.com**, where you can share your stories. This venue will allow you to communicate with me as well. Let me know what worked. I would like to know if there are additional questions that you would like to have answered. If you are still struggling, let me know what is missing or what is not working. If there are sections, or themes in this book that are not clear, let me know. If there are concepts or theories that you hear about that you feel are relevant to this conversation, I welcome your contribution. I will take all this into consideration for future editions of this book.

Please visit the
USE YOUR MIND TO HEAL YOUR BODY
website at:

www.UseMindBody.com

Today, we are at the early stages of an informational campaign. If you share with colleagues around the water cooler at work or with your family at the dinner table that your pain was/is psychologically induced, you may raise a few eyebrows. However, being able to discuss and articulate these concepts is important. To be clear, I am not suggesting that you need to convince, or defend anything. External validation is no substitute for your inner knowing. There will certainly be moments when *not* discussing the subject is more appropriate. There will also be moments where sharing your trials, tribulations, understanding and victories may be most helpful. Your story may save someone years of pain. Sharing and contributing to others not only provides an invaluable service, it also eliminates self-doubt and paves the road to recovery for millions of people searching for a better way to recover from needless suffering.

Glinda, The Good Witch, to Dorothy:
You don't need to be helped any longer.
You've always had the power.

Dorothy:
I have?

Scarecrow:
Then why didn't you tell her before?

Glinda:
Because she wouldn't have believed me.
She had to learn it for herself.

—The Wizard of Oz

RECOMMENDED REFERENCES

BOOKS ON PSYCHOSOMATIC PAIN

Healing Back Pain by John E. Sarno, MD

Easy to read and understand, powerfully outlines the psychology, physiology and treatment of mindbody disorders. Recommended for anyone interested in Dr. Sarno's work, especially back pain sufferers.

The Mindbody Prescription by John E. Sarno, MD

Dr. Sarno advances his theory pointing at rage, not anger, as a principle emotion from which pain serves to distract our attention. With comprehensive attention to "equivalents" to back pain, I recommend this book to people suffering from the various other emotionally induced maladies such as shoulder, hip, knee pain, digestive disorders, headaches, allergies and skin disorders.

The Divided Mind by John E. Sarno, MD

With a comprehensive history of psychosomatic medicine, extensive coverage of why the medical profession ignores mindbody concepts, and six chapters each written by different medical doctors treating TMS, I especially recommend this book to doctors and healthcare professionals.

USE YOUR MIND TO HEAL YOUR BODY

Pathways to Pain Relief by Eric Sherman, Psy.D, (the psychotherapist who treated me) and Frances Sommer Anderson, Ph.D

This is a powerfully effective and insightful book that vividly details the psychotherapeutic process particularly with respect to psychosomatic treatment.

Books on Meditation and Spirituality

A Course in Miracles, Foundation for Inner Peace

A Return to Love by Marianne Williamson

Medical Doctors who Treat Mindbody Disorders

Ira G. Rashbaum, MD
NYU Langone Medical Center
240 East 38th Street, New York, NY 10016
(212) 263-6477
E-mail: ira.rashbaum@nyumc.org

Dr. Rashbaum is clinical professor of physical medicine and rehabilitation at New York University School of Medicine and an attending physiatrist at the Rusk Institute of Rehabilitation Medicine. He trained directly under and worked with Dr. Sarno from 1992 to 2012 and has been diagnosing and treating patients with psychosomatic pain disorders for over twenty years.

WEBSITES

The Tension Myositis Syndrome Wiki
Compiled by former patients who have become or are in the process of becoming pain-free using treatment first diagnosed by Dr. Sarno, this site provides excellent resources including support forums, practitioner directories, Q & As with experts, and a Structured Education Program. This is a content-rich online resource:
http://www.tmswiki.org

Psychologic Disorders Association
The Psychophysiologic Disorders Association is non-profit organization dedicated to educating medical practitioners, mental health professionals, and the public about psychophysiologic disorders (PPD) and increasing the availability of practitioners skilled in their treatment:
http://www.ppdassociation.org

USE YOUR MIND TO HEAL YOUR BODY

RECENT RESEARCH IN THE FIELD OF MINDBODY MEDICINE

There is a rapidly expanding body of scientific research substantiating and supporting Dr. Sarno's mindbody diagnosis and therapeutic approach.

Researchers at the above-referenced *Tension Myositis Syndrome Wiki* [http://www.tmswiki.org] have compiled an extensive listing of hundreds of books, presentations and peer-reviewed articles published in the world's most reputable and prestigious medical journals.

Their data is divided into two parts:

The **Annotated Bibliography** "created for researchers and lay people alike, contains summaries, links to abstracts and full texts of articles, information about authors, information about related research, and other helpful information about the most important research relevant to TMS." A list of these articles is included here, without summaries.

The Master Bibliography is "intended primarily for researchers as a comprehensive list of all articles cited in books, articles, or presentations about TMS."

Please note that, as with all *Wikis*, content is under active development. The entries below were referenced on November 30, 2012 from:

http://www.tmswiki.org/ppd/Medical_Evidence

LISTINGS FROM *THE TMS WIKI* "ANNOTATED BIBLIOGRAPHY:"

Kerns, Robert; Hoffman, Benson. "Meta-analysis of psychological interventions for chronic back pain." *Health Psychology*, 2007. 26(1),1-9.

Raspe, Heiner; Hueppe, Angelika; Neuhauser, Hannelore. "Back pain, a communicable disease?" *International Journal of Epidemiology*, 2008. 37;69-74.

Bigos, SJ; Battie, MC; Spengler, DM; et al "A longitudinal, prospective study of industrial back injury reporting." *Clinical Orthopaedics and Related Research*. June 1992, 279:21-34.

Schofferman, J, et al. "Childhood psychological trauma correlates with unsuccessful lumbar spine surgery." *Spine*. 1992 Jun; Vol. 17(6 Suppl):S138-44.

Rashbaum, Ira; Sarno, John. "Psychosomatic Concepts in Chronic Pain." *Archives of Physical Medicine and Rehabilitation*. 2003. Volume 84, Supplement 1:S76-S80.

Koo, J and Lebwohl, A. "Psychodermatology: The Mind and Skin Connection." *American Family Physician*, 2001. 64:1873-1878.

Bailer, JC. "The Powerful Placebo and the Wizard of Oz." *New England Journal of Medicine*. 2001. 344:1630-1632.

Bass, Christopher; Peveler, Robert; House, Allen. "Somatoform Disorders: Severe Psychiatric Illnesses Neglected by Psychiatrists." *British Journal of Psychiatry*. 2008 Vol. 179, 11-14.

Eisenberger, NI; Lieberman Matthew D. "Why rejection hurts: a common neural alarm system for physical and social pain." *Arthritis & Rheumatism*. May 2002; 46(5):1333-1343

Strigo, Irina A, et al. "Major Depressive Disorder is Associated with Altered Functional Brain Response During Anticipation and Processing of Heat Pain." *General Psychiatry*. November 2008,65(11);1275-1284.

Derbyshire, SWG, et al. "Cerebral activation during hypnotically induced and imagined pain." *Neuroimage*. September 2004,23(1);392-401.

Bailey, KM, et al. "Treatments addressing pain-related fear and anxiety in patients with chronic musculoskeletal pain: a preliminary review." *Cognitive Behavior Therapy*. March 2010; 39(1):46-63.

Burns, J, et al. "Arousal of negative emotions and symptom-specific reactivity in chronic low back pain patients." *Emotion*: May 2006;6(2):309-19.

Burns, J, et al. "Effects of anger suppression on pain severity and pain behaviors among chronic pain patients: evaluation of an ironic process model." *Health Psychology.* September 2008;27(5):645-52.

Moseley, G, et al. "Thinking about movement hurts: the effect of motor imagery on pain and swelling in people with chronic arm pain." *Arthritis and Rheumatology.* May 15, 2008; 59(5):623-31.

Okifuji, A, et al. "Stress and psychophysiological dysregulation in patients with fibromyalgia syndrome." *Applied Psychophysiology and Biofeedback.* June 27, 2002 (2):129-41.

McBeth, J, et al. "Moderation of psychosocial risk factors through dysfunction of the hypothalamic-pituitary-adrenal stress axis in the onset of chronic widespread musculoskeletal pain: findings of a population-based prospective cohort study." *Arthritis and Rheumatism* January 2007; 56(1):360-71.

Nahit, E, et al. "The influence of work related psychosocial factors and psychological distress on regional musculoskeletal pain: a study of newly employed workers." *Journal of Rheumatology.* June 2001; 28(6):1378-84.

Ghiadoni, Lorenzo; Donald Ann E; Cropley, Mark; et al. "Mental Stress Induces Transient Endothelial Dysfunction in Humans." *Circulation.* 2000 Vol. 102: 2473-2478.

Gracely, Richard H; Petzke, Frank; Wolf, Julie M; and Clauw, Daniel J. "Functional Magnetic Resonance Imaging Evidence of Augmented Pain Processing in Fibromyalgia." *Arthritis & Rheumatism.* May 2002. 46(5):1333–1343.

Abeles, Aryeh M; Pillinger, Michael, H; Solitar, Bruce, M; and Abeles, Micha. "Narrative Review: The Pathophysiology of Fibromyalgia." *Annals of Internal Medicine.* May 15, 2007. 46(10): 727-735.

Burgmer, Markus, et al. "Decreased Gray Matter Volumes in the Cingulo-Frontal Cortex and the Amygdala in Patients with Fibromyalgia." *Psychosomatic Medicine.* 2009. Vol. 71:566-573.

Derbyshire, S, et al. "Fibromyalgia pain and its modulation by hypnotic and non-hypnotic suggestion: an fMRI analysis." *European Journal of Pain.* May 2009; 13(5):542-50. Epub. July 23, 2008.

Alvares, T, et al. "[Fibromyalgia: interfaces to RSI and considerations about work etiology.]" (In Portuguese) *Ciencia & Saude coletiva.* May 2010; 15(3):803-12.

Cedradhi, C, et al. "Fibromyalgia: a randomized, controlled trial of a treatment programme based on self management." *Annals of the Rheumatic Diseases.* March 2004; 63(3):290-6.

Buskila, D, et al. "A painful train of events: increased prevalence of fibromyalgia in survivors of a major train crash." *Clinical and Experimental Rheumatology* September-October 2009;27(5 Suppl 56):S79-85.

Fink, P, et al. "One single diagnosis, bodily distress syndrome, succeeded to capture 10 diagnostic categories of functional somatic syndromes and somatoform disorders." *Journal of Psychosomatic Research.* 2010 May; 68(5):415-26.

Hsu, Michael; Schubiner, Lumley, Howard, Mark; Stracks, John; et al. "Sustained Pain Reduction Through Affective Self-awareness in Fibromyalgia: A Randomized Controlled Trial." *Journal of Internal Medicine.* October 2010, 25, Issue 10, pp 1064-1070.

Larkin, M. "Carpal Tunnel Syndrome Study Stirs Controversy." *The Lancet,* June 16, 2001. 357 (9272).

Adkins, S; Figler, R. "Hip Pain in Athletes." *American Family Physician,* 2000. 61:2109-2118.

Jones, G, et al. "Predicting the onset of knee pain: results from a 2-year prospective study of new workers." *Annals of Rheumatic Disease.* 2007 Mar;66(3):400-6. Epub 2006 Aug 25.

Berry, D; Pennebaker, JW. "Nonverbal and verbal emotional expression and health." *Psychotherapy and Psychosomatics.* 59(1), 1993, 11-19.

Smyth, Joshua. "Effects of Writing About Stressful Experiences on Symptom Reduction in Patients With Asthma or Rheumatoid Arthritis: A Randomized Trial." *Journal of the American Medical Association.* April 14, 1999. 281(14):1304-1309.

Zeidan, Fadel; Gordon, Nakia; et al. "The Effects of Brief Mindfulness Meditation Training on Experimentally Induced Pain." *The Journal of Pain.* Published online 23 October 2009.

Craig, A, et al. "The effects of slow breathing on affective responses to pain stimuli: An experimental study." *Journal of the International Association for the Study of Pain.* Published online January 15, 2010.

Kabat-Zinn, J, et al. "The clinical use of mindfulness meditation for the self-regulation of chronic pain." *Journal of Behavioral Medicine.* 1985 Jun; 8(2):163-90.

Grossman, P, et al. "Mindfulness-based stress reduction and health benefits. A meta-analysis." *Journal of Psychosomatic Research.* 57, Issue 1 , Pages 35-43, July 2004.

Kaplan, KH, et al. "The impact of a meditation-based stress reduction program on fibromyalgia." *General Hospital Psychiatry.* Gen. Hosp. Psychiatry. September 1993;15(5):284-9.

Grossman, P, et al. "Mindfulness training as an intervention for fibromyalgia: evidence of postintervention and 3-year follow-up benefits in well-being." *Psychotherapy and Psychosomatics.* 2007; Vol. 76(4):226-33.

Smith, BW, et al. "A pilot study comparing the effects of mindfulness-based and cognitive behavioral stress reduction." *The Journal of Alternative Medicine.* April 2008; 14(3):251-8.

Esterling, BA; Antoni, MH; et al. "Emotional disclosure through writing or speaking modulates latent Epstein-Barr virus antibody titers." *Journal of Consulting and Clinical Psychology.* 1994, 62(1): 130-140.

Sadlier, M, et al. "Tinnitus rehabilitation: a mindfulness meditation cognitive behavioural therapy approach." *The Journal of Laryngology and Ontology.* 2008 Jan;122(1):31-7. Epub 2007 Apr 23.

Davidson, R, et al. "Alterations in Brain and Immune Function Produced by Mindfulness Meditation." *Psychosomatic Medicine* 65:564-570 (2003).

Schrader, H; Obelienniene, D; Bovim, G; Surkiene, D; Mickeviciene, D; Miseviciene, L; et al. "Natural evolution of late whiplash syndrome outside the medicolegal context." *Lancet.* 1996, 347.

Ferrari, R; Kwan, O; Russell, AS; Schrader, H; Pearce, JMS. "The best approach to the problem of whiplash? One ticket to Lithuania, please." *Clin. Exp. Rheumatol.* May-June 1999. 17(3):321-6.

Castro, WH; Meyer, SJ; Becke, ME; Nentwig, CG; Hein; MF; Ercan, BL; et al. "No stress - no whiplash? Prevalence of "whiplash" symptoms following exposure to a placebo rear-end collision." *International Journal of Legal Medicine.* 2001, 114: 316-22.

Obelieniene, Diana; Schrader, Harald; Bovim, Gunnar; Misevic, Irena, Sand, Trond. "Pain after whiplash: a prospective controlled inception cohort study." *Journal of Neurological Neurosurgical Psychiatry.* 1999. Vol.66: 279–283.

THANK YOU DR. SARNO PROJECT

When Dr. Sarno retired in April 2012, several colleagues and former patients of his handcrafted a book containing a collection of acknowledgment letters and presented this tribute as a token of appreciation to him. I was fortunate enough to have my letter included as part of what became the "Thank you Dr. Sarno Project." Read other letters at www.thankyoudrsarno.org

Dear Dr. Sarno:

I am so pleased to have this opportunity to thank you, acknowledge you, and honor you.

Under your care and treatment I was returned to health and it seems only fitting for me to make this information as available as possible so that others can also have the opportunity to heal from psychosomatic pain.

Several years ago I limped into your office with excruciating lower back pain that severely impacted the quality of my life for 15 years. In the two years prior to meeting you, I could not walk properly, run or dance without burning pain. I tried physical therapy, chiropractors, acupuncture, deep tissue massage, and even hanging upside down from my ankles for hours (inversion therapy). None of that worked. Then, NYC's most prominent surgeons recommended back surgery and they had MRIs and X-rays to back-up their recommendations. As a last chance effort to avoid surgery, I went to see you. After working with you and Dr. Eric Sherman, one of your gifted psychotherapists, my pain disappeared. Treatment took less than a year and I have now been pain-free for over ten years.

Since I am a Professional Engineer, I was able to see the disk abnormalities on the MRIs. It was therefore very difficult to not subscribe to the physical diagnosis given to me by so many doctors. In the face of my skepticism you held your ground and declared that while the pain is real, the source is not the disk but the mind. It was in your certainty that I found the courage to discover, confront and come to terms with painful emotions from which the pain served to distract me. When it was no longer necessary to be distracted from these emotions, the pain ceased to serve a function and went away.

I thank you for your courage to stand in the face of little to no agreement from the medical establishment. I acknowledge you for being a doctor who, early on in your medical practice, told the truth to yourself and others when your patients did not get better using popular and lucrative (to doctors and medical and insurance companies) treatments—and then found a way to get your patients better. I honor you for distinguishing a new paradigm for the treatment of chronic pain.

The Collins Dictionary defines genius as "a person with exceptional ability, especially of a highly original kind; distinctive spirit or creative nature; a person exerting great influence." Collins uses the example, "Mozart's musical genius." Future generations will no doubt use the phrase, "Dr. Sarno's medical genius." In every sense of the word, you are a genius. I am honored and fortunate to have been treated by you and to know you.

With deep appreciation and abiding respect,

Steve Conenna

ENDNOTES

[1] Proverb from India
[2] J. E. Sarno, *Healing Back Pain* (New York: Warner Books, 1991), 89.
[3] J. E. Sarno, *Mind Over Back Pain* (New York: William Morrow & Co., 1984).
[4] J. E. Sarno, *Healing Back Pain* 8.
[5] J. E. Sarno, *The Mindbody Prescription* (New York: Warner Books, 1999) 11.
[6] J. E. Sarno, *The Mindbody Prescription* 141.
[7] J.E. Sarno, *The Mindbody Prescription* 36.
[8] J. E. Sarno, *The Divided Mind* (New York: Harper Collins, 2006) 130.
[9] J. E. Sarno, *The Divided Mind* (New York: Harper Collins, 2006) 129.
[10] J.E. Sarno, *The Divided Mind* 130.
[11] J. E. Sarno, *The Mindbody Prescription* xxi.
[12] J. E. Sarno, *Healing Back Pain* 95.
[13] J. E. Sarno, *The Divided Mind* 2.
[14] J. E. Sarno, *The Mindbody Prescription* 35.
[15] J. E. Sarno, *The Mindbody Prescription* 108.

[16] J. E. Sarno, *The Divided Mind* 15-31.
[17] J. E. Sarno, *Healing Back Pain* 48.
[18] M. C. Jensen, et al, *Magnetic resonance imaging of the lumbar spine in people without back pain*, <u>New England Journal of Medicine</u> 331 (1994): 69-73.
[19] J. E. Sarno, *The Mindbody Prescription* 142.
[20] J. E. Sarno, *The Divided Mind* 11.
[21] J. E. Sarno, *The Mindbody Prescription* 141.
[22] J. E. Sarno, *The Mindbody Prescription* xiv.
[23] J. E. Sarno, *The Mindbody Prescription* 162.
[24] J. E. Sarno, *The Mindbody Prescription* 108.
[25] J. E. Sarno, *Healing Back Pain* 75.
[26] J. E. Sarno, *The Mindbody Prescription* 108.
[27] J. E. Sarno, *The Divided Mind* 87.
[28] J.E. Sarno, *The Divided Mind* 31.
[29] *The American Heritage® Dictionary of the English Language* (Fourth Edition copyright ©2000 by Houghton Mifflin Company, 2009).
[30] J.E. Sarno, *The Mindbody Prescription* 142.
[31] J.E. Sarno, *The Divided Mind* 136.
[32] J.E. Sarno, *Healing Back Pain* 82.
[33] J.E. Sarno, *The Divided Mind* 143-145.
[34] J.E. Sarno, *Healing Back Pain* xii.
[35] In recent years several articles have questioned the value of certain types of back surgery and the possible overuse of spine surgery:

- Jerome Groopman, *A Knife in the Back – Is surgery the best approach to chronic back pain?* The New Yorker (April 8, 2002).
- Reed Abelson and Melody Peterson, *An Operation to Ease Back Pain Bolsters the Bottom Line, Too*, The New York Times (December 31, 2003).
- Richard A. Deyo, MD, et al, *Spinal-Fusion Surgery—The Case for Restraint*, The New England Journal of Medicine (February 12, 2004).
- James N. Weinstein, DO, MSc., *Surgical vs. Nonoperative Treatment for Lumbar Disk Herniation*, Journal of the American Medical Association (JAMA) (November 22/29, 2006) Vol 296, No. 20.
- Reed Abelson, *The Spine as Profit Center*, The New York Times (December 30, 2006).

[36] J.E. Sarno, *The Mindbody Prescription* xxvi.

[37] J.E. Sarno, *The Divided Mind* 4.

[38] http://www.tmswiki.org/ppd/Medical_Evidence, Referenced November 30, 2012

[39] J.E. Sarno, *The Divided Mind* 3.

[40] *Relieving Pain in America: A Blueprint for Transforming Prevention, Care, Education, and Research* (IOM, Institute of Medicine, 2011), 2.

[41] *Relieving Pain in America*, 19.

NOTES:

NOTES:

Please visit the
USE YOUR MIND TO HEAL YOUR BODY
website at:

www.UseMindBody.com

I am very interested in hearing from you.

- Get questions answered
- Share your success story
- Provide feedback about the book
- Order additional copies

Made in the USA
San Bernardino, CA
29 November 2018